Head Injury
And Its
Complications

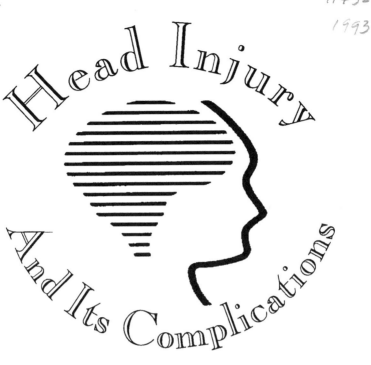

Head Injury And Its Complications

Edited by
James L. Stone, M.D.
Divisions of Neurosurgery, Neurology
and Electroencephalography
Cook County Hospital
and
Departments of Neurology and Neurological Surgery
University of Illinois Hospital
Chicago, Illinois

PMA PUBLISHING CORP.
Costa Mesa, California

To Michelle, Jasmine and Jett

**NOTICE: The editors, contributors, and publisher of this work have made every effort
to ensure that the drug dosage schedules and/or procedures are accurate and in
accord with the standards accepted at the time of publication . Readers are
cautioned, however, to check the product information sheet included in the package of
each drug they plan to administer. This is particularly important in regard to new or
infrequently used drugs. The publisher is not responsible for any errors of fact or
omissions in this book.**

Library of Congress Cataloging in Publication Data
Head injury and its complications / edited by James L. Stone.
     p.   cm.
    Includes bibliographical references and index.
    ISBN 1-56262-008-8 : $50.00
    1. Brain — Wounds and injuries — Treatment.   2. Brain — Wounds and
injuries — Complications.   1. Stone, James L. (James Leland), 1948-

    [DNLM: 1. Brain Injuries — complications.   WL 354 H4323]
RD594.H394   1992
617.5'1044 — dc20
DNLM/DLC
for Library of Congress   92-49059
                                                  CIP

Printed in the United States of America

List of Contributors

Albino Bricolo, M.D., Department of Neurosurgery, University Hospital, Verona, Italy.

Robert M. Crowell, M.D., Neurosurgical Service, Massachusetts General Hospital and Harvard Medical School, Boston, Massachusetts.

George R. Cybulski, M.D., Division of Neurosurgery, Cook County and Northwestern Memorial Hospital, Chicago, Illinois.

Anthony DiGianfilippo, M.D., Department of Neurosurgery, Presbyterian St. Luke's Hospital, Chicago, Illinois.

Howard M. Eisenberg, M.D., Division of Neurosurgery, University of Texas Medical Branch, Galveston, Texas.

Ramsis F. Ghaly, M.D., Divisions of Neurosurgery and Neuroanesthesia, Cook County Hospital, Chicago, Illinois.

Frederic A. Gibbs, M.D., Department of Neurology and Electroencephalography, University of Illinois Hospital, Chicago, Illinois.

Felicia C. Goldstein, Ph.D., Department of Neurology, Neurobehavioral Program, Emory University School of Medicine, Atlanta, Georgia.

John R. Hughes, Ph.D., M.D., Department of Neurology and Electroencephalography, University of Illinois Hospital, Chicago, Illinois.

Harvey S. Levin, Ph.D., Division of Neurosurgery, University of Texas Medical Branch, Galveston, Texas.

Robert A. Moody, M.D., Section of Neurosurgery, The Guthrie Clinic, Sayre, Pennsylvania.

J. Paul Muizelaar, Ph.D., M.D., Division of Neurosurgery, Medical College of Virginia, Richmond, Virginia.

Seigo Nagao, M.D., Department of Neurological Surgery, Kagawa Medical School, Kagawa, Japan.

Walter D. Obrist, Ph.D., Department of Neurosurgery, University of Pennsylvania Hospital, Philadelphia, Pennsylvania.

James L. Stone, M.D., Divisions of Neurosurgery, Neurology and Electroencephalography, Cook County Hospital, and Departments of Neurology and Neurological Surgery, University of Illinois Hospital, Chicago, Illinois.

Oscar Sugar, Ph.D., M.D., Department of Neurological Surgery, University of Illinois Hospital, Chicago, Illinois and the University of California at San Diego.

Contents

Contents

Introduction

Remarkable progress has been made in the understanding and treatment of head injuries over the past ten to twenty years. Not only have we seen the development and wide application of diagnostic techniques for timely identification of intracranial pathology, but we have also become aware of a multitude of detrimental factors and secondary insults, some preventable, to the already injured brain. Perhaps the most important factors are airway control and prompt delivery to a neurosurgically equipped trauma center. Computerized tomographic brain scans almost always detect surgically significant intracranial lesions. The value of a large craniotomy and careful post-operative monitoring has become clear. In addition to the clinical examination, a number of newer physiological tools, including intracranial pressure monitoring, cortical and brainstem evoked potentials, and cerebral blood flow studies, are now at our disposal to monitor the care of this most challenging group of patients. These clinical tools may also be strong prognostic indicators. Seizures, neurobehavioral and medicolegal consequences of the injury must be confronted. This volume addresses these challenging issues and points to areas for future investigation.

The editor is especially grateful to Drs. Robert Moody and Oscar Sugar for stimulating an intense interest in head injury, and to Ms. Ernestine Daniels for devoted assistance with manuscript preparation.

FOREWORD

Oscar Sugar, Ph.D., M.D.

Evaluations into geological strata dating many thousands of years before the present era attest to the ubiquity of head injury in man. A few of the uncovered skulls appear to have had trepanation associated with healed fractures. The motivation behind the other early craniotomies remains obscure; suggestions offered in explanation include release of pressure or blood clots or evil spirits. In any case, paleontology indicates the length of the history and widespread occurrence of head (and brain?) injury. Certainly in the centuries which have followed, with "civilization" (and its attendant wars, population stresses, and increased industrialization, multistoried buildings, and self-propelled vehicles) the incidence of head and brain injuries has multiplied manyfold. The task of the doctor and his/her allies is to minimize the incapacity of the injured person; and it is to this burden that Dr. Stone and his colleagues have devoted this book.

The initial chapter deals with the pathophysiological principles which dictate the management of patients with acute head trauma. Rapid transport to a trauma center, rather than to the nearest hospital, is emphasized along with the need for a "team" to care for the whole patient. Careful and repeated monitoring and prompt action in the case of a questionable finding can make significant improvement in outcome of head injury, especially if intracranial blood clots can be cared for within 4 hours of injury. Sections of text also deal with cerebral perfusion pressure as well as intracranial pressures — how to monitor them and change them. Controversies about intracranial pressure monitoring and the use of steroids are discussed, especially with recommendations on the reduction of raised intracranial pressure.

The specific surgical technique used by Dr. Stone and one of his mentors, Dr. Robert Moody, have withstood the test of time in one of the busiest trauma centers in the United States, at the Cook County Hospital in Chicago. Diagnosis of the exact locus of a suspected blood clot is assisted by computerized tomography; and before that was available, by angiograms. However, when the patient appears to be deteriorating with evidence of brainstem compression, exploratory burr holes are not to be delayed by waiting for the radiographic tests. The value of temporal lobectomy, usually partial, is emphasized, and the authors have not hesitated to remove portions of the dominant temporal lobe when necessary, ordinarily sparing the speech regions.

Peculiarities of head injury in children are shown to be related to age groups, subdivided into those who have just been born, those under age 2, and after fontanelle closure. A variant of the Glasgow Coma Scale, an Infant Coma Score, is offered by Drs. Cybulski and Stone as an aid in evaluation in that age category. The apparent greater resistance of the child's brain to injury as compared to adults is a subject of investigation, and meaningful changes in treatment can be based on this.

The chapter on cerebral blood flow and metabolism following severe head injury represents a forward step in the understanding of the events in the "black box" representing the traumatized head and its contents. Just how the monitoring of cerebral flow may help in the practical problems faced by those who care for these patients is only hinted at initially, but the importance of knowledge of the relation between cerebral metabolism and blood flow is stressed. Considerable detail is given in the portion of the book on measurements of blood flow, and oxygen and carbon dioxide differences in arteries and veins. Later in this chapter, the purposes and values of studying cerebral flow are presented, with particular emphasis on evaluation of various therapeutic regimens.

Muizelaar and Obrist were able to show a statistically valid trend for higher blood flow with better coma scores; but in individual patients, it has not been possible to relate cerebral blood flow and clinical condition. There appears to be no purpose in carrying out such tests beyond 24 hours after head injury, and it appears that cerebral blood flow and Glasgow Coma Score are related only in the early period after head injury. Caution with very vigorous hyperventilation must be exercised. The benefit of mannitol in increasing cerebral blood flow in animals has been reported. This implies that it may also be valuable in treating humans with head injury. Ischemia, the authors conclude, plays a distinct but very small role in determining outcome after severe head injury. Comparisons are made between the vasospasm which has been observed after head injury and that which follows aneurysmal rupture; one sometimes forgets that the most common cause of subarachnoid bleeding is head injury.

While mannitol may be valuable in adults with head injury by increasing blood flow, it may carry dangerous increase in intracranial pressure in children. The authors discuss the uses of mannitol and of hyperventilation in children with head injury. The relationship between cerebral blood flow and intracranial pressure remains un-clarified.

The reasons behind the impairment of metabolic autoregulation and of vascular autoregulation are still unclear, and exactly what is to be done about it is equally a problem at present.

The detection of electrical impulses from the head (and neck) in patients with head injury is described by Stone and his associates among whom are long-time leading figures in this field: F.A. Gibbs and John R. Hughes. The first chapter deals with the electroencephalogram proper; the second, sensory evoked potentials. The electroencephalogram in acute trauma lacks reliability and should not be used to make decisions in the ordering of tests such as computerized tomograms and angiograms; local trauma to the scalp can make it unwise to attempt to study exactly the part underlying the blow to the head.

Standard electroencephalography has been carried out in patients with head injuries over many years. However, such refinements as computerized spectral arrays may be used in prediction of outcome in patients with midbrain syndromes and coma. Early seizures increase the mortality, so detection and therapy for possible epileptogenic areas may improve the outcome. It may be that treatment can be started when study reveals electrographic seizures of which the staff has been prewarned, and this may prevent some complications, especially if the patient is deliberately paralyzed with pharmacological agents or is in barbiturate coma.

Evoked potentials produced by stimulation of peripheral nerves, visual and auditory pathways can give clinically useful data in evaluation of the central nervous system after head injury, particularly in unconscious patients. Changes in temporally sequential observations are often of prognostic significance. Evoked potentials may permit assessment of patients in barbiturate coma and after allied induced techniques to control raised intracranial pressure. Physiological evaluation of central nervous system lesions may also be estimated by using evoked potentials; even concomitant injuries such as dorsal root avulsions can be associated with changes in evoked sensory potentials.

A major problem associated with head injury has to do with post-traumatic epilepsy. Whether or not to give prophylactic anticonvulsants in the hope of preventing seizures is currently unsettled. John Hughes has taken into account the timing, incidence, and clinical characteristics of this disorder. A broad discussion is given to the medico-legal aspects of head injury—a subject of much importance in practical medicine but often ignored or glossed over. Of particular interest in this regard is the occurrence of antisocial behavior (especially violent criminal acts) and psychiatric aberrations in patients with post-traumatic epilepsy. His advice, particularly pertinent to the electroencephalographer as legal witness, might also apply to the neurosurgeon or neurologist as witness.

The closing chapter on neurobehavioral outcome of injuries to the brain is by psychologists Goldstein and Levin and neurosurgeon Howard Eisenberg. A variety of psychologic tests dealing with "intelligence," memory, attention, and language disturbance have been applied to patients recovering from closed-head injury. Tests for behavioral change are less readily quantified and need expansion to allow therapists to deal more effectively with patients who have disturbances in insight, motivation, somatic complaints, emotional outbursts, etc. The authors are impressed by the paucity of data concerning the effects of head injury in "older" patients.

Overall, this volume on head injury has much value in current treatment and in the understanding of patients with head injury. It points to lines of research to be used in future development of care, since we are so deficient in our ability to prevent head injury—which should be the ultimate goal of all medical care; that is, prevention to make treatment unnecessary. Pending the attainment of this unreachable goal, as "the Man from La Mancha" would have it, we rely on books such as this to guide our practice and also show the directions to be taken to improve the outcome of head injury.

ABBREVIATIONS

AEP: Auditory evoked potential (long latency)
ANOVA: Analysis of variance
ASDH: Acute subdural hematoma
AVDO2: Arteriovenous (jugular) difference of oxygen content
BAEP: Brainstem auditory evoked potential
BBB: Blood-brain barrier
CBF: Cerebral blood flow
CBV: Cerebral blood volume
CCT: Central conduction time
CHI: Closed head injury
CMRO2: Cerebral metabolic rate of oxygen consumption (= CBF x AVDO2)
CNS: Central nervous system
CPAP: Continuous positive airway pressure
CPP: Cerebral perfusion pressure (= MAP minus ICP)
CSA: Compressed spectral array EEG
CSF: Cerebrospinal fluid
CT: Computerized tomographic brain scan
CTT: Central transmission (conduction) time
CVP: Central venous pressure
CVR: Cerebral vascular resistance
Cz: Vertex region electrode
DAI: Diffuse axonal injury
dB: decibels
dBpeSPL: Decibels peak sound pressure level
dBSPL: Decibels sound pressure level
DCR: Direct cortical response
ECochG: Electrocochleography
EEG: Electroencephalogram
EP: Evoked potential
EVD: External ventricular drainage
GCS: Glasgow Coma Score
GOS: Glasgow Outcome Score
ICP: Intracranial pressure

ICS: Infant Coma Score
ICU: Intensive care unit
IM: Intramuscular
IMV: Intermittent mandatory ventilation
IPL: Interpeak latency
IQ: Intelligence quotient
IV: Intravenous
kg: Kilogram
LOC: Loss of consciousness
MAP: Mean arterial pressure
MBAEP: Modified brainstem auditory evoked potential
mCi: Millicurie
mCi/l: Millicurie per liter
MEP: Multimodality evoked potential
min: Minute
ml: Milliliter
MLR: Middle latency auditory responses
mm: Millimeter
mmHg: Millimeters of mercury
mmH$_2$O: Millimeters of water
MRI: Magnetic resonance image brain scan
PEEP: Positive end-expiratory pressure
PET: Positron emission tomographic brain scan
PLED: Periodic lateralized epileptiform discharge (in EEG)
PSVEP: Pattern-shift visual evoked potential
PTA: Post-traumatic amnesia
PTE: Post-traumatic epilepsy
PVI: Pressure volume index
SD: Standard deviation
SE: Standard error
SEP: Somatosensory evoked potential
SSEP: Short latency somatosensory evoked potential
VEP: Visual evoked potential
vol%: Volume percent
WAIS: Wechsler adult intelligence scale

Chapter 1

Acute Head Trauma Management and Pathophysiological Principles

James L. Stone, Ramsis F. Ghaly, Anthony Di Gianfilippo, and Robert M. Crowell

INTRODUCTION

Trauma is a major health problem in the United States with high mortality and morbidity rate. It ranks third as a cause of death and is considered the number one killer of people between one and forty-four years of age. Injury to the head constitutes a pivotal health problem because associated brain damage makes the largest contribution to ultimate outcome, accounting for two thirds of deaths. About 500,000 cases of head injury occur annually in the United States and head injury is found in 75% of patients suffering other injuries. The leading causes of head trauma are transportation accidents, violence, and falls. Roughly two thirds of the total number of fatal head injuries are caused by vehicular accidents, and one third is the result of homicide or suicide. One in every twelve deaths results from injuries such as falls. In urban areas such as Chicago, up to 96% of fatal wounds are due to interpersonal violence [5,10,21,33,34].

The overall head injury mortality rate is about 50,000 deaths per year in the United States. At least two thirds of all deaths due to head injury occur prior to hospital inpatient care. The incidence of head injury in males is three times that of females, and the male mortality rate from head injury is three to four times greater than the female mortality rate. Peak mortality is highest among young adults and the elderly. Of all head injury patients discharged alive, about 10% are discharged with significant neurologic impairment and 1% in a vegetative state [10,21,23,33,47].

1

2   *Stone, Ghaly, Di Gianfilippo, and Crowell*

The last decade has seen improvement in the outcome of head-injured patients attributed to a careful understanding of current principles in head injury management. These methods include: (1) rapid transport of the injured patient, (2) prompt airway control with arterial blood oxygenation and avoidance of hypercarbia, (3) early diagnosis and management of mass lesions, (4) prevention and early treatment of secondary insults, (5) fluid and electrolyte balance, (6) control of intracranial pressure (ICP) and maintenance of adequate cerebral perfusion pressure (CPP), (7) continuous assessment of the patient's cardiopulmonary and neurological status, (8) frequent follow-up with computerized tomographic (CT) scans, especially in the early days after injury, (8) provision of nutritional support, and (10) a comprehensive rehabilitation program.

CLASSIFICATION OF HEAD INJURY

Head injury may be simply classified into focal and diffuse brain injuries.

Focal Injuries

Focal injuries are localized to a limited area of the brain and are the result of mechanical injury produced at the time of immediate or secondary impacts. Contact phenomena include scalp, skull, meningeal, and localized brain injury. Types of focal injuries are: (1) intracranial hematoma – subdural, epidural, and intraparenchymal, (2) contusion – bruising of the brain, (3) laceration – frank disruption of brain tissue, and (4) a variable degree of brain swelling. Focal injuries account for approximately 50% of all hospital admissions for head injury, depending on the population studied. Focal injuries can become manifest immediately after the initial trauma or may appear hours or days after injury [11,12].

Diffuse or Generalized Brain Injuries

Diffuse or generalized brain injuries are felt to be the result of widespread shearing or rotational forces and are often secondary to vehicular injury (Figure 1.1). Simple concussion is a mild form of diffuse injury defined as a transient loss of cerebral function or memory lapse after injury with no permanent brain damage. A more serious consequence of diffuse injury has come to be called diffuse axonal injury (DAI). In this condition, physical disruption of axons is found in many regions of the brain associated with deep brain hemorrhages. This type of injury not infrequently leads to a comatose state and is a common cause of persistent neurological disability in survivors. Diffuse head injuries probably account for about 50% of hospitalized head-injured patients and about one third of head injury deaths [11,12].

It has been shown that vehicular injuries more commonly produce diffuse injuries which may require only ICP monitor placement. Conversely, blunt assault or falls more commonly produce focal intracranial hematomas requiring surgery [4,21,30].

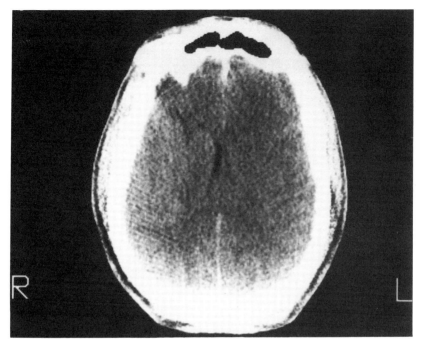

Figure 1.1. Plain CT scan of the brain. Sulci are not seen and both frontal horns are effaced. Note lucency in both frontal regions. An example of diffuse brain injury with a suggestion of increased intracranial pressure. Subarachnoid hemorrhage is also believed to be present. If the patient is comatose (GCS < 8), ICP monitoring may aid medical management and give an early warning of delayed hemorrhage or further swelling.

Secondary Insults

Secondary insults resulting from trauma can be either intracranial or systemic. Secondary intracranial injury is often associated with ischemia, local or generalized cerebral edema, and elevated ICP. Contusional hemorrhages may enlarge over hours or days, possibly related to coagulopathy. Impairment of cerebral autoregulation may be a factor leading to secondary brain injury [9,30]. Autoregulation is the ability of cerebral arterioles to maintain a constant cerebral blood flow (CBF) across the range of mean arterial blood pressure from 50 to 150 mmHg.

Systemic Causes of Brain Injury

Systemic causes of brain injury include: hypercarbia, hypoxia, hypotension, anemia, electrolyte imbalance, hyperthermia, or other metabolic disturbances including coagulopathy of disseminated intravascular type and release of catecholamines. The occurrence of secondary insults obviously correlates with higher mortality and morbidity rates. Prevention and early treatment of these insults can dramatically improve the outcome of patients with severe head injury. Unfortunately, any combination of focal, diffuse, or secondary injury can occur and complicate an individual head injury case [3,9,13,30,38].

Head trauma can also be divided into open or closed injury, depending on whether a dural tear, cerebrospinal fluid leak, or communication with the outside environment is present. Skull fractures (linear, depressed, compound) are important correlates of impact injury and brain damage. In addition, the fracture itself may require surgical treatment.

EMERGENCY MANAGEMENT AT THE SCENE AND EN ROUTE

Rapid transport of the head injured patient directly to a trauma center capable of providing early aggressive medical and surgical treatment has been shown to significantly improve outcome [2,4,9,16,30,40,41]. The patient is usually transferred by ambulance or helicopter. In an urban setting it is advisable for the resuscitation team to spend minimal time at the scene. Radio contact to the trauma center is established en route to aid monitoring the patient's condition prior to arrival. In some parts of the world, the physician and the pilot fly to the scene of the injury to avoid delay in treatment [6]. The patient should be transported in the supine position with the cervical spine fully stabilized. Approximately 5% to 15% of severely head-injured patients have an associated cervical spine injury [16,21]. A patent airway, ventilation, and intravenous lines must be maintained and oxygen administered as necessary. Intubation may be needed at the scene or en route. Hypoxia and hypotension can develop almost immediately after injury due to a variety of causes.

Hypotension should be controlled immediately in order to maintain the cerebral perfusion pressure (CPP). Prompt control of any external bleeding by pressure dressings may be necessary. Blood loss from scalp lacerations can be substantial and underestimated. Infants and toddlers can lose significant amounts of blood intracranially and go into shock. Intravenous fluids are given at adult rates of 83 to 120 cc/hr or more through large bore (16g) catheters and blood is drawn for later typing and crossing. If systolic blood pressure falls below 100 mmHg, medical measures for shock are indicated.

The patient's *vital signs should be monitored* frequently, and neurological assessment performed every five minutes during transport to the trauma center. Neurological assessment should consist primarily of the level of consciousness, Glasgow Coma Score (GCS) (see Table 1.1), pupillary size, and pupillary reactivity to light. A thorough survey of other body systems must also be performed.

IN THE TRAUMA CENTER

A *complete resuscitative team* must be available at the trauma center. This team consists of a general surgeon, neurosurgeon, orthopedic surgeon, and anesthesiolo-

Table 1.1. Glasgow Coma Scale [44]	
Eye Opening	
4	Spontaneous
3	To verbal command
2	To pain
1	None
Motor Response	
6	Obeys command
5	Localizes pain
4	Normal flexion-withdrawal
3	Abnormal flexion (decortication)
2	Extension (decerebration)
1	None
Verbal Response	
5	Oriented and converses
4	Disoriented and converses
3	Inappropriate words
2	Incomprehensible sounds
1	None
Score	
15	Normal
13-14	Mildly abnormal
9-12	Moderately abnormal
3- 8	Severely abnormal

gist to evaluate the patient for possible multiple injuries and to carry out the appropriate emergency measures.

In the trauma unit, a *definitive airway* via endotracheal intubation, nasotracheal intubation, cricothyroidotomy, or tracheostomy should be placed in the unconscious patient and artificial ventilation started. Nasal intubation is often preferred in patients with possible neck injury and cervical instability. The indications for assisted ventilation include: apnea, irregular respiratory pattern, respiratory rate greater than 40 breaths per minute or less than 10 per minute, tidal volume less than 1.5 cc/kg, vital capacity below 1L, $PaCO_2$ level greater than 45 mmHg, and PaO_2 level less than 70 mmHg. The PaO_2 level should be maintained above 100 mmHg, the $PaCO_2$ level should be initially maintained between 25 mmHg and 30 mmHg, and the tidal volume should be maintained at 10-15 cc/kg. Continuous positive airway pressure (CPAP), intermittent mandatory ventilation (IMV), positive end-expiratory pressure (PEEP), and controlled ventilation are the most common methods used to provide respiratory support [1].

Shock

Shock following multiple trauma must be rapidly assessed and treated. The most frequent hemodynamic abnormalities encountered in patients with severe head injury are elevated systolic blood pressure, tachycardia with a rate greater than 120 beats per minute, and increased cardiac output. Intracranial hypertension may be accompanied by systemic hypertension and bradycardia but it is a late event (Cushing response). Hypovolemic hypotension following head injury in the older child or adult is rare in the absence of blood loss from scalp lacerations and multiple trauma (chest, abdomen, long bones). About 90% of head trauma patients with multiple injuries develop anemia defined as hematocrit value less than 30% [9]. This should not be overlooked because it may further exacerbate ischemic complications from other causes.

Continuous Monitoring

Continuous monitoring of *arterial blood pressure*, and frequent measurements of *central venous pressure* and *cardiac output* (occasionally pulmonary wedge pressure measurement may be necessary) are *essential to maintain adequate cerebral perfusion*. A *Foley catheter* should be inserted and complete assessment of fluid intake and output made periodically. A nasotracheal or nasogastric tube should not be inserted if there is a severe fracture of the maxilla or frontal base or a penetrating neck injury. *Peritoneal lavage* is frequently required as internal bleeding may otherwise escape notice, especially in comatose or obtunded patients. Routine laboratory tests, blood and urine toxicology screen, tetanus prophylaxis, and x-rays of skull, cervical spine, and chest are performed in the trauma unit. Mannitol (1 gm/kg) is given for pronounced obtundation or suspected herniation. Naloxone hydrochloride (possible narcotic overdose if pupils are small), Dextrose 50 and anticonvulsants are medications that may need to be administered shortly after the assessment. Steroids are no longer routinely used in severe head injury and have not been shown to be effective [9,10,16]. However, the steroid methylprednisolone, in large doses for 24 hours has recently been shown to be beneficial for spinal cord injury [6].

Neurological Evaluation

A neurological evaluation is made in the trauma unit by a neurosurgeon. The physician must give special consideration to the following aspects of the neurological examination: the patient's *highest level of consciousness and arousability, Glasgow Coma Score, pupillary size and reactivity to light, and stereotypic motor posturing (decerebration or decortication). Other neurologic signs* of brain stem dysfunction include abnormal oculo-vestibular reflex (cold calorics), corneal, cough, and gag reflexes. Vigorous Doll's eye (oculo-cephalic) testing is not advisable unless cervical spine films are normal, but caloric testing may be performed if the tympanic membranes are visualized and intact. Lateralizing signs include cranial nerve dysfunction (6th nerve palsy may be non-specific), unilateral deep tendon reflex changes, paresis, paralysis, or unilateral sensory loss (in those patients alert enough for sensory testing). Anisocoria in an obtunded patient, with or without fixation to light, is highly localized and indicative of ipsilateral tentorial herniation unless orbital or eye trauma is present. Cerebellar, lower cranial nerve, or respiratory abnormalities may be found with posterior fossa injuries. A head trauma patient's pupils should rarely be artificially dilated, otherwise an important diagnostic parameter will be lost.

The GCS does not always correlate with the patient's neurological injury. The level of consciousness cannot be reliably evaluated in patients with shock, hypoxia, intoxication, or postictal state. A retrospective study showed that 90% of awake patients who later deteriorated had early symptoms such as persistent severe headache, agitation, and respiratory rate greater than 20 breaths per minute [26].

Physical findings with neurological implications that should attract a trauma physician's attention include CSF leakage (rhinorrhea or otorrhea), ear or nasal bleeding, subconjunctival hemorrhage, periorbital edema, scalp lacerations, and tenderness or bruises over the scalp. A rigid neck may indicate cervical spine injury, occipital fracture, subarachnoid hemorrhage, or tonsillar herniation. Tenderness over the spine with associated spinal cord or cauda equina injury may not be clearly apparent in an unconscious patient. Direct transfer to a specialized unit with personnel skilled in caring for head-injured patients will obviously reduce delay in definitive care and improve the outcome of these patients. A CT scanner should be available within minutes and operating rooms must be rapidly available. A complete physical and neurological examination is performed as soon as possible. Patients with multiple systemic injuries remain in the trauma unit with close follow-up by the neurosurgical service if a head injury exists or is suspected. An injury to the spine also requires immediate neurosurgical or orthopedic attention and immobilization.

Emergency Radiologic Studies

Emergency radiologic studies include portable *skull x-rays* in all severe head-injured patients (GCS ≤ 8) provided that there is no delay in the patient's management. Anteroposterior, Towne's, and cross-table lateral skull views are strongly recommended in patients with history of altered mental status, loss of consciousness of more than 10 minutes, or focal neurological deficit. Also patients with scalp lacerations, gunshot, or penetrating wounds to the head require plain skull films.

A CT scan should be obtained, as soon as the patient's condition is stabilized if intracranial pathology is thought possible. The following conditions warrant an emergency, non-contrast CT brain scan: focal neurologic signs, mental status changes, severe headache, prominent linear, diastatic, or depressed skull fracture. It may be necessary to reduce patient agitation in order to obtain an adequate CT brain scan. Intubated patients may be given morphine sulfate or pancuronium bromide with careful monitoring. Naloxone sulfate reversal may be given but may precipitate withdrawal in addicts. Diazepam may be judiciously used in small increments but respirations must be carefully monitored.

In situations where a CT scan is unavailable, a cerebral angiogram or ventriculography may be performed. The laterality and approximate location of a lesion may be ascertained and shift of the midline structures detected. *Emergency cerebral angiography* is indicated in cases of penetrating injury to the neck or skull base, injuries in relation to a major intracranial venous sinus, or atypical parenchymal hemorrhages where an aneurysm or malformation may be suspected.

An *osmotic diuretic* such as Mannitol is required in obtunded patients with suspected increased ICP or tentorial herniation as determined by clinical examination and/or CT scan. However, in the acute setting, Mannitol is only used to buy time for an emergency diagnostic procedure such as CT scan or in those about to undergo emergency craniotomy. The effect of Mannitol may be temporary and deceiving in the face of an expanding intracranial mass lesion. The patient should remain at bed rest with head elevated thirty degrees in the normotensive individual. Other measures to acutely control ICP are hyperventilation, barbiturates, and surgical evacuation of intracranial hematomas (see below).

EMERGENCY SURGERY

Intracranial hematomas can be defined as acute (less than 24 hours after injury), early subacute (within first three days), subacute, or chronic (greater than 10 days to two weeks after injury) [42]. Early diagnosis and prompt evacuation of the mass lesion may markedly improve the outcome in these patients (Figures 1.2 to 1.4). Delay in treatment of intracranial hemorrhage is a common avoidable factor leading to death [2,3,9,30,40,41]. A report showed marked improvement in mortality rate (from 90% to 30%) for patients with acute subdural hematoma operated upon *within 4 hours of injury* [40]. The quality of life in survivors was also significantly better for those operated soon after injury. Delay in definitive treatment of mass lesions results from delay in referring patients for definitive neurosurgical care, lack of awareness of delayed post-traumatic intracerebral hematomas, or misdiagnosis. Neurological symptoms and signs may be inaccurately attributed to acute alcoholism, cerebrovascular accidents, psychiatric or behavioral disturbances [9,41]. Delayed traumatic intracerebral hemorrhage after trauma can occur within hours or days after injury. The frontal and temporal lobes are the most common sites. A higher incidence of delayed hemorrhage is seen in patients suffering from hypoxia, systemic hypertension, or coagulopathy.

Measures to *combat delayed treatment* or misdiagnosis include: rapid transport to an experienced trauma center with available neurosurgical coverage, 24 hours per day CT brain scan capability, and close monitoring of all patients admitted with head injury [41]. The presence of focal neurological deficits, changes in mental status, or severe headache should arouse suspicion of an intracranial mass lesion. An intracranial lesion not detected on an initial CT brain scan may sometimes be found on a repeat scan. Patients with depressed or linear *skull fractures* that cross meningeal vascular grooves or venous sinuses are at particular risk to develop an intracranial hematoma. In a retrospective study, about 50% of patients who later severely deteriorated had a skull fracture and developed an intracranial hematoma [26].

An emergency temporal burr hole for partial evacuation of blood clot may be performed in patients with pupillary signs of uncal or temporal lobe herniation when

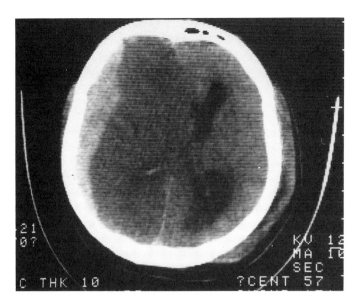

Figure 1.2. Plain CT scan. Massive acute subdural hematoma. Note lucency of the hemisphere underlying the clot and 1 to 2 cm midline shift. Dilatation of the contralateral ventricular system indicates third ventricle or aqueduct obliteration related to clinical signs of herniation in the patient. Emergency surgery is indicated.

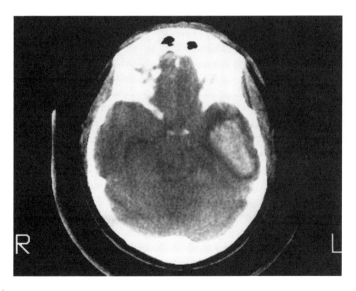

Figure 1.3. Plain CT scan. A large anterior temporal lobe contusional hematoma is apparent. Note the near-absence of basal cisterns and enlargement of contralateral temporal horn. A small amount of low density area (edema) surrounds the clot. The patient slept when left alone and had a hemiparesis. Emergency surgery is indicated.

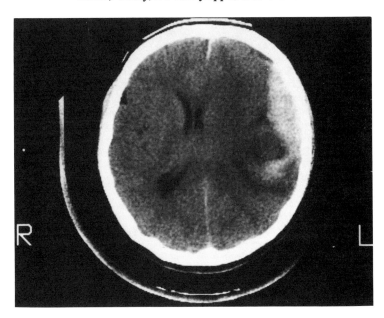

Figure 1.4. Plain CT scan. A frontoparietal, lens-shaped extradural hematoma is apparent with underlying small, mixed density contusional hemorrhage. The frontal horns are shifted approximately 1 cm across the midline and the frontal horn on the side of hematoma is effaced. A small amount of blood is noted along the falx. Emergency surgery is indicated.

delay for CT scan is deemed dangerous. Burr holes and small craniectomies performed in the trauma unit or operating room have recently again been advocated for rapid diagnosis and temporizing treatment of suspected traumatic intracranial space-occupying hematomas. This is the situation when even a modest time delay may be fatal [2,42]. We perform an emergency temporal trephination on the side of the larger pupil or the first pupil to dilate. A dilated pupil is one equal to or greater than 6 millimeters. The trephination procedure is only done for non-penetrating head injuries where one or both dilated pupils fail to come down 10 to 15 minutes after IV mannitol and hyperventilation. If a clot is detected, it often extrudes under pressure and the patient is brought for immediate generous craniotomy. A CT brain scan or diagnostic cerebral angiography is performed immediately following craniotomy or in those patients with negative temporal trephinations to identify other possible lesions [42]. Pupillary asymmetry may be unreliable if the patient has had recent seizures, orbital trauma, a Horner's syndrome, or the rare direct midbrain or third nerve injury.

The *need for surgery* is usually determined by the patient's clinical status, degree of mass effect, and location of mass lesion on CT scan. A temporal mass lesion is potentially more serious than a frontal or parietal mass lesion due to proximity of the medial temporal lobe to the midbrain. Patients with significant midline shift (5 mm across the midline) require immediate consideration for surgery. The best results are obtained with a wide operative exposure extended to the frontotemporal base.

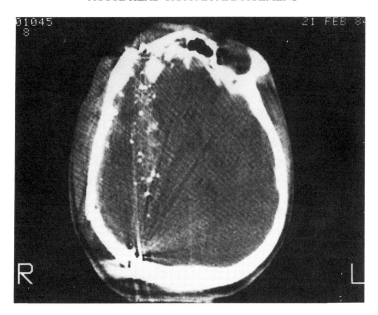

Figure 1.5. Plain CT scan. A gunshot wound crossed the skull and brain from frontal to occipital regions. Note comminution and depressed bone and bullet fragments along the track of the missile. The brain is diffusely swollen and coagulopathy was clinically apparent. The patient was brain dead within one hour of admission.

This allows for complete evacuation of the hematoma and devitalized contused brain tissue. A contralateral ICP monitor may be placed at the time of surgery. Reaccumulation of blood, brain swelling, and infection are possible postoperative complications.

In *missile injuries* such as gunshots, brain damage often results from the direct effect of the missile and also from a tremendous amount of kinetic (blast effect) energy transmitted intracranially (Figure 1.5.). Concurrent with tissue penetration, intracranial pressure may rise and cause further brain damage and herniation. Progressive cerebral swelling may account for a rapid deterioration of neurological function shortly after the injury. The resulting brain injury may include a varying combination of contusion, laceration, hemorrhage, and brain edema along the missile track including tangential and distant areas. Gunshot wounds of the brain may also cause major arterial or venous sinus injury, traumatic aneurysm, and cavernous-carotid fistula. Injury to the dominant transverse sinus, posterior two-thirds of the sagittal sinus, or vein of Galen may be fatal. Moreover, rupture of intracranial vessels may produce significant intra- and/or extraparenchymal hematoma. Expansion of a hematoma may also contribute to later deterioration of neurological function as compensatory mechanisms fail. Cerebral edema may be progressive over several days.

Missile-injured patients require immediate resuscitation including the above-mentioned emergency measures. Operative management may include: (1) debridement of entrance as well as exit wounds, (2) evacuation of intracranial hematoma and necrotic contused brain, (3) removal of accessible bone and missile fragments without causing further damage, (4) ICP monitoring, and (5) meticulous dura and scalp closure.

Missile wounds outside CNS should not be overlooked and must be strongly suspected if unexplained hypotension exists. Patients with a penetrating injury to the brain may later develop intracranial infection such as meningitis or abscess formation, particularly in the presence of CSF leakage, retained bone fragments, necrotic brain tissue, or dural opening. Consequently, prophylactic use of broad spectrum antibiotics is recommended. Calvarial gunshot wounds must be debrided in those patients who show cerebral or brain stem functioning.

SUBSEQUENT MANAGEMENT

Anticonvulsant therapy is indicated if a generalized or focal seizure occurs at the time of injury or later. Phenytoin (Dilantin) is the drug of choice for seizures in the immediate post-traumatic period. The loading dose is 10 to 15 mg/kg with the intravenous rate not to exceed 50 mg/minute. The patient should be observed for bradycardia or hypotension and blood levels monitored. Diazepam 0.1 to 0.3 mg/kg IV will usually temporarily stop status epilepticus, but respirations must be carefully watched.

Prophylactic anticonvulsant therapy is indicated in head-injured patients with focal neurologic deficits or CT confirmed contusion, and extra- or intra-axial space occupying hematomas. Foreign body deposition within brain tissue as in missile injuries, depressed skull fractures, or an intracranial infective process also warrant anticonvulsants.

The maintenance dose of Dilantin is 5 mg/kg per day as a single dose or divided into three equal doses. Phenobarbital (loading 10 to 15 mg/kg, maintenance 5 mg/kg/day) may be administered if a second drug is necessary to control seizures. Respiratory depression may result with higher doses of barbiturates. Pentobarbital coma may also be applied for generalized seizure control (see below under ICP control). Carbamazepine (Tegretol) is a very useful anticonvulsant for focal or secondary generalized seizures, however it must be given orally or by nasogastric tube. At least one drug is continued for one year post injury with gradual tapering of the dose over several months thereafter if there has been no seizure. A normal electroencephalogram (EEG) should ideally be obtained prior to discontinuing the anticonvulsant. Patients with spikes or sharp waves on follow-up sleep EEGs will probably require anticonvulsants indefinitely.

Treatment of the patient with traumatic CSF leak (rhinorrhea or otorrhea) is controversial and includes penicillin, broad spectrum antibiotic coverage or no antibiotics. We treat with meningeal doses of intravenous ampicillin and keep our patients flat in bed until 2 to 3 days after leakage has ceased. If the leakage persists after 3 to 5 days, lumbar drainage of CSF may be tried. If there is no resolution within 10 days to two weeks, surgery is indicated. About 90% of those with rhinorrhea and nearly all with otorrhea resolve without continued fluid leakage or bouts of meningitis necessitating reparative surgery.

In general, head trauma patients do not require *prophylactic antibiotics*. Nevertheless, patients with penetrating wounds, scalp lacerations over obvious skull fractures, skull fractures through the air sinuses, or macerated, contaminated scalp wounds should receive prophylactic antibiotics. Placement of an ICP monitoring device may require prophylactic antibiotics and ideally the device should be changed or removed after 72 hours to reduce the chance of infection [32]. A central venous or radial arterial catheter should ideally be changed or removed after 72 hours to reduce the possibilities of infection.

Patients in coma need *nutritional support* either by tube feeding or hyperalimentation. This may be started 3 to 4 days after injury as the patient's general condition permits. An average of 50% increase in the resting metabolic expenditure has been reported with severe head injury. The major determinant of caloric requirement appears to be the severity of neurologic injury [8,15]. Oral feeding can be started as soon as the patient's condition improves. Hyperalimentation may be given in patients where tube feeding is not appropriate (e.g., paralytic ileus, abdominal surgery).

Fluid and electrolyte disturbances represent another major problem in head-injured patients [25]. The causes include inappropriate secretion of antidiuretic hormone, inappropriate administration of IV fluids or mannitol effects, and less frequently, diabetes insipidus. Appropriate measures should be taken promptly to combat any fluid and electrolyte imbalance. Resuscitation fluids should contain glucose and sodium. Inappropriate secretion of antidiuretic hormone is treated with fluid restriction or sodium replacement if severe (Na < 120 mg%). Diabetes insipidus, on the other hand, is treated with fluid replacement and vasopressin or desmopressin administration if fluid intake cannot be matched with urine output.

Regarding pulmonary care, once the patient can ventilate independently and protect his airway, he is taken off the respirator and observed on CPAP. The patient is extubated if chest x-ray and arterial blood gases do not indicate a problem. An intensive rehabilitation program beginning with bedside physical therapy should be started as soon as possible.

PATHOPHYSIOLOGICAL CONSIDERATIONS

Cerebral Perfusion Pressure and Intracranial Pressure

The *normal CPP* ranges from 80 to 90 mmHg and is equal to the MAP minus ICP. (Mean arterial pressure, MAP, equals one third of pulse pressure plus diastolic pressure.) For example, if systemic blood pressure is 120/80, pulse pressure is 40; MAP = 40/3 + 80 = 93; if ICP is 15 mmHg, CPP = 93 - 15 = 78.

An adequate CPP of at least 50 to 60 mmHg must be maintained by blood pressure elevation and/or reduction of elevated ICP. Inadequate CPP in trauma patients may lead to cerebral ischemia and possibly cerebral infarction. Most neurosurgeons consider an ICP of 16 to 20 mmHg elevated and an indication for aggressive medical management [1,3,25,27,30,39]. Uncontrolled ICP greater than 20 mmHg is clearly associated with a poorer outcome [9,25,27,28,29].

Systolic hypotension and CT scan evidence of ventricular asymmetry or shift, if present within 24 hours of injury, will increase the incidence of ICP exceeding 30 mmHg over the next few days. There is a higher incidence of elevated ICP (> 30 mmHg) in patients with *absence of basal cisterns* on CT brain scan. But elevated ICP has also been reported in patients with normal basal cisterns [22,45].

Elevated ICP

Elevated ICP can result from a variety of causes. These include *cerebral hyperemia, hypoxia, hyponatremia or water intoxication, sepsis, seizures, and hypertension*. Cerebral hyperemia may be defined as a condition in which cerebral blood flow (ml/100gm of brain/minute) is increased to a degree greater than that required for tissue metabolism. There is a higher incidence of cerebral hyperemia in patients whose CT scan shows diffuse brain edema or swelling on admission. Furthermore, one study showed that about 70% of patients with an elevated ICP (> 20 mmHg) had acute cerebral hyperemia. High ICP was found in 57% of cases with hyperemia in contrast to only 23% with reduced cerebral blood flow [35]. Hyperventilation would appear to be the treatment of choice for increased ICP associated with hyperemia.

Other causes of high ICP include *delayed brain edema or swelling, delayed traumatic intracerebral hematomas, increase in the size* of a pre-existing intracranial mass lesion, and *hydrocephalus*. Impairment of the blood brain barrier and cerebral autoregulation may play a role in elevating ICP in severely head-injured patients.

Not yet resolved is the issue of the indications for ICP monitoring in head-injured patients. One approach is to monitor ICP in all patients where elevated ICP is likely to develop and may require surgical or medical intervention. In these situations, ICP monitoring is used as a guide for timely therapy. Elevated ICP is a good indication for a repeat CT scan. Clinical status and vital signs may be unreliable indicators of ICP. In addition, ICP monitoring can be of prognostic value and can provide an early warning of an expanding or delayed intracranial mass lesion or a postoperative clot.

Patients at risk to develop elevated ICP include: (1) patients with temporal or frontal lobe contusions, (2) patients with GCS scores of 8 or less following resuscitation, (3) patients with abnormal motor posturing, (4) patients with abnormal CT brain scan, e.g., presence of mass lesion, shift, or compressed basal cisterns, (5) patients with normal CT scan but with unexplained neurological deterioration, and (6) patients with systolic hypotension. ICP recording will not be helpful in patients who are considered untreatable due to severity of their intracranial or systemic injuries or lack of brain stem function [16,22,25,27,29,30,32].

ICP Monitoring Systems

There are four commonly used ICP monitoring systems. These are: (1) *Intraventricular catheter* which provides the most accurate recording of ICP and permits drainage of CSF. CSF drainage may at times effectively control ICP, especially in hydrocephalic conditions. However, it is occasionally difficult to cannulate the ventricles and penetration of the brain is required. (2) *Subarachnoid or subdural bolt*: A twist drill hole is made in the skull and dura is opened. The bolt is easy to place and is fairly reliable but fluid damping and occlusion of the bolt may occur. (3) *Subdural catheter*: The bolt is relatively easy to place and is preferred by some surgeons. Frequent irrigation may be necessary to maintain patency. (4) *Extradural sensors* have more calibration problems but lower infection rate and they may be kept in place for longer periods of time. The recent fine intraparenchymal fiberoptic (Camino) sensor is gaining popularity. All of these ICP monitors may be placed in the intensive care unit (ICU) or operating room. Ventriculostomy is relatively contraindicated in cases of disseminated intravascular coagulopathy, platelet count below 100,000, or prothrombin time greater than twice normal [43].

Complications of ICP monitoring with ventriculostomy include infection which occurs in about 8% of cases and hemorrhage [32]. The incidence of infection may be reduced when a closed drainage system is used. Intraventricular catheter, subdural, or subarachnoid devices are replaced or moved to a new site every 3 days and the duration of monitor placement is reduced. The ICP monitor should be discontinued when sustained ICP consistently remains below 18 to 20 mmHg.

Management of High ICP

Recent reports have shown that early aggressive therapy of elevated ICP more often results in good control of ICP. The higher the level at which control of ICP is attempted, the more difficult it is to lower the ICP. Initial ICP of 40 to 60 mmHg or more is usually poorly controlled and death or vegetative outcome is virtually assured [9,25,28,29,39]. Elevated, uncontrolled ICP represents the cause of death in over 50% of severely head-injured patients who die and ICP correlates strongly with poor mortality and morbidity rates [25,27,29,39]. The incidence rate of elevated ICP is greatest in patients with intracranial clots, especially acute subdural hematoma [29,35]. Over half of this group show persistent or recurrent elevated ICP even after evacuation of the mass lesion [29,42].

Measures should be taken to aid jugular venous drainage. An endotracheal tube or collar should not be taped too firmly around a patients neck, and a straight head position with 30 degree head elevation is maintained in comatose patients. Head-injured patients with increased CVP or raised intrathoracic pressure from venous causes often present with ICP problems.

Sustained systemic hypertension (MAP greater than 30% of normal mean value) should be treated with close observation of the CPP in severely head-injured patients. A beta adrenergic blocker, such as propranolol, may be used to titrate blood pressure and heart rate. Vasodilators, such as hydralazine, trimethaphan, or nitroglycerin, may be used to treat systemic hypertension. Sodium nitroprusside may give excessive cerebrovascular dilatation and increased ICP [25]. Careful monitoring of MAP and ICP should be carried out in order to maintain adequate CPP above 50 to 60 mmHg.

The *acute management of elevated ICP* includes the following: (1) Hyperventilation to maintain the $PaCO_2$ between 25 to 30 mmHg is the initial treatment of choice to reduce elevated ICP. (2) Mannitol (20%, 1.0 gm/kg) is given intravenously as bolus or continuously. Fluid and electrolyte balance should be checked regularly. Serum osmolarity should be maintained below 315 mosm. (3) Immediate evacuation of a significant intracranial mass lesion if present. (4) The patient's head should be *elevated 30 degrees* unless otherwise contraindicated by systemic hypotension or cervical spine injury. (5) Half-normal saline with glucose is given as maintenance fluid in adults with serum sodium, potassium, and osmolarity maintained within normal limits. (6) Muscular paralyzing agents such as pancuronium bromide (0.1 mg/kg) may be necessary in actively decerebrating patients. (7) Sodium thiopental infusion (3 mg/kg), lidocaine (1 to 1.5 mg/kg IV), or ambu bagging may be performed prior to endotracheal suctioning or intubation. (8) Ventricular cerebrospinal fluid drainage may also be tried to control ICP. (9) Therapeutic barbiturate coma is begun only if all other measures to control ICP (> 30 mmHg) are problematic or have failed. The assumption is that lowered cerebral metabolic requirements result in decreased cerebral blood volume and increased tolerance of ischemia. Pentobarbital, 10 mg/kg/hr IV infusion, is given over the first four hours and the 1.6 mg/kg/hr IV infusion is given thereafter [39]. Close monitoring of cardiac output and arterial blood pressure is required. A burst suppression pattern on EEG reflects a physiologic dosage. High doses of barbiturates can successfully lower the elevated ICP and this appears to benefit an occasional patient, but it does not clearly improve the overall mortality. CPP must be carefully monitored and blood pressure well maintained. Problems with barbiturates may include hypothermia, pneumonia, and loss of the neurological examination [1,25].

PaO_2-$PaCO_2$ Levels

It is widely accepted that hypoxia and hypercarbia are by far the most common preventable events following head trauma. Hypoxemia ($PO_2 < 70$ mmHg) may develop soon after injury [3,9,16,38]. This situation calls for prompt intubation and mechanical ventilation. The reported mortality rate of patients with hypoxemia is 50%, compared to 24% in patients without any systemic insult [12]. Hypercarbia ($PaCO_2 > 40$ mmHg) is associated with cerebral vasodilation, increased cerebral blood volume, and increased ICP. Hypercarbia is frequently found in trauma patients who are too obtunded to protect their airway. There appears to be a marked outcome improvement in patients treated with controlled hyperventilation.

Hypoxia following head injury may be due to poor cerebral perfusion secondary to increased ICP or more commonly peripheral causes such as pulmonary aspiration or infection, pulmonary edema, or chest trauma. Other causes include disseminated intravascular coagulopathy, fat embolism, and iatrogenic sources including incorrect placement of an endotracheal tube, pneumothorax following subclavian puncture, hematoma in the neck following angiography, fractured ribs following resuscitation, and intravenous fluid overload.

Arterial-jugular bulb oxygen content difference (AVDO2) or the cerebral oxygen extraction fraction has been measured to aid medical management of head injury patients. Samples of cerebral venous blood are obtained by inserting a catheter in the internal jugular vein superior to the jugular bulb. Any arterial site can be used to obtain the arterial samples. From hemoglobin oxygen saturation calculation, rough estimation of a hyperemic or ischemic intracranial state may be obtained as well as the overall cerebral metabolic rate of oxygen consumption (CMRO2). Cerebral hyperemia can be treated by hyperventilation and ischemic conditions treated with continuous infusion of mannitol (i.e., 500 cc/8 hrs) [1,36]. Near-infrared light spectrum and positron emission tomography (PET) scanning have recently been applied to further study the oxidative metabolic status of the brain [7].

Cerebral Blood Flow Monitoring in Head Trauma

CBF represents 15% of cardiac output and is normally 50 to 60 ml/100g/minute. A noninvasive technique to measure CBF in head trauma patients is performed by the inhalation or intravenous administration of [133]Xenon [31,36,37]. Regional radio-activity is monitored by eight scintillation detectors placed over each hemisphere. Flow values are calculated with bicompartmental as well as infinity methods. Results are usually available within twenty minutes. The level of CBF is remarkably stable throughout a wide spectrum of activity except in extreme situations such as seizures or vasospasm. There is a critical value for CBF under which basic metabolism cannot be maintained and neuronal cells disintegrate. It has been shown in monkeys that ischemic infarction occurs immediately with flow levels of 7 ml/100g/minute, after 2 to 3 hours with flow levels of 10 to 12 ml/100g/minute, and with sustained flows of 18 ml/100g/minute [20].

CBF measurement allows assessment of the adequacy of blood flow to the brain as well as providing a means of detecting and preventing low CBF which may lead to ischemia and infarction. Increasing CBF in this situation has been shown to improve the CMRO2 and neurological function in selected head-injured patients. Ischemia may develop with normal, increased, or low blood pressure and it may be dangerous to reduce blood pressure without knowledge of CBF or CPP.

Ischemia does play a role in determining the clinical status and outcome of severe head-injured patients. Recent reports indicate that CBF measurement is helpful in predicting outcome [31,35,36,37]. There is a correlation between CBF and clinical status during the initial post-injury phase. The level of blood flow to a hemisphere correlates with the clinical condition and Glasgow motor score. Poor outcome (dead or vegetative) can be expected in patients with very low CBF.

CBF measurement can also be used to evaluate cerebral autoregulation as well as cerebrovascular reactivity to changes in $PaCO_2$. It should be recalled that CPP = CBF/cerebral vascular resistance. Most cerebrovascular reactivity is confined to the arterial system. Larger arterioles are important in regulating the flow of blood to the brain capillary bed at which exchange of gases, nutrition, and metabolites takes place. Arteriolar diameter can be decreased 20% or increased 65% by hypocarbia or hypercarbia, respectively, leading to a 36% decrease or 172% increase in arterial blood volume. Mannitol infusion is also known to increase arteriolar diameter and cerebral blood flow [31]. In patients with impaired autoregulation, a rapid increase in systolic blood pressure can cause extravasation of blood and possibly promote brain edema. Autoregulation is often impaired in head-injured patients with low motor Glasgow Coma Scores [31,36].

In normal individuals, there is a positive correlation between local brain activity, local oxygen consumption, and regional blood flow. In head-injured patients, $CMRO_2$ is decreased proportionately with the depth of coma and CBF may be abnormally low (matching), normal, or abnormally (mismatching) [31,36].

CBF is increased in situations of high metabolic (mainly oxygen and glucose) demand, such as seizures or hyperthermia, and reduced in cases of low metabolic demand, as in barbiturate coma or hypothermia [31].

Abnormally high CBF (hyperemia) or abnormally low CBF may occur in head trauma patients. Furthermore, these abnormalities may be focal or generalized. Seventy-five comatose patients were studied within 72 hours of injury [36]. It was shown that 55% of the cases developed hyperemia and 45% developed a reduction in CBF. Hyperemia was strongly associated with elevated ICP.

Electrophysiology in Head Trauma Management

Scalp recorded evoked potentials (EP) are computer averaged responses of the nervous system to a specific sensory stimulus, either auditory, visual, or somatosensory. EP monitoring is a noninvasive procedure which can be performed at the bedside. In recent years, neurologists and neurosurgeons have applied EPs to the intensive care and operating room settings. EPs have been used to serially monitor the neurologic status of severely head-injured patients, specifically those with GCS scores equal or less than 8 [14,24].

The *indications of EP monitoring in acute head injury* are: (1) to test neuronal pathway function and determine the severity or localization of injury, (2) to detect insults early enough to avert potentially disastrous consequences, e.g., brain stem ischemia detected by auditory evoked response and cerebral ischemia detected by somatosensory evoked response, (3) to guide the efficacy of medical management, (4) to confirm a diagnosis, e.g., by differentiating coma caused by intrinsic brain stem lesions from toxic/metabolic or cerebral cause, (5) to assess brain function in patients with chemical paralysis or barbiturate coma, since their neurological status cannot be followed solely by the standard clinical basis, and (6) to predict outcome with an accuracy rate above 90% within the first 72 hours after injury [14,24]. The routine EEG is important in diagnosis and management of post-traumatic seizure disorders. Computerized, compressed EEG spectral analysis has also been used in the ICU and may aid in prediction of post-traumatic coma [24]. Routine EEG and cerebral blood flow methods are extremely important in the confirmation of brain death.

OUTCOME

The *Glasgow Outcome Scale* (GOS) developed by Jennett and Bond is often used to classify the outcome of head trauma patients [17,44]. This is a 5-point classification which includes: (1) *Good Recovery* – patient is totally independent and able to return to previous level of employment, (2) *Moderate Disability* – patient is independent and may be able to regain some form of occupation with mild physical or behavioral impairment, (3) *Severe Disability* – such as hemiplegia, aphasia, or dementia, the patient is dependent on others for daily activities, (4) *Permanent Vegetative State* – patient does not follow any commands or communicate, is not responsive to changes in the environment but spontaneous eye opening and sleep/wake cycles may return, and (5) *Death*. This classification can be reduced to a *3-point classification* which includes: (1) *Functional outcome* – good recovery and moderate disability, (2) *Severe disability and vegetative state*, and (3) *Death*. The majority of deaths from severe head injury occur during the first month post injury. By three months, two thirds of head-injured patients have attained their final outcome status and by *six months*, 95% of patients have attained their final outcome status [18,19]. Further significant improvement in the quality of life can occur as late as two to three years post injury, but they seldom change the Glasgow outcome level. The outcome of head trauma patients correlates will with the initial post-resuscitation GCS score, and in particular the motor score. Eye opening is also of prognostic value in the first few days following injury and may indicate a better outcome.

Factors associated with poor outcome include advanced age, low socioeconomic class, previous CNS damage, pre-existing medical disorders, gunshot wounds, high speed acceleration-deceleration injury, depressed skull fracture, penetrating wounds, intracranial mass lesion, GCS score of 8 or below, abnormal motor posture, dilated fixed pupils, impaired or absent eye movement, signs of brain stem dysfunction, abnormal CT scan findings (e.g., absent basal cisterns), early secondary insults, moderate to severely abnormal auditory or somatosensory evoked responses and associated serious extracranial conditions [3,14,22,35,38,29,45].

Among the *complications* that commonly occur in head trauma patients and aggravate the course of the illness are: respiratory, cardiovascular, or renal disorders, gastrointestinal bleeding, disseminated intravascular coagulopathy, CNS infections, and endocrine dysfunction including diabetes insipidus and inappropriate secretion of antidiuretic hormone. Prevention or early diagnosis and aggressive treatment are required to combat these complications.

Delayed enlargement of the lateral ventricles or cerebral sulci indicates cerebral atrophy. This frequently occurs within the first three months after severe injury and is associated with a higher incidence of severe disability. The finding of ataxia and dysarthria is higher in patients with an enlarged fourth ventricle [47]. Enlargement of ventricles (if associated with persistent or intermittently increased ICP) may require a ventriculoperitoneal shunting procedure.

The *post-traumatic syndrome* is a common complication seen in patients following minor or moderate head injury. It is a complex of somatic, psychophysiological, and behavioral complaints usually presenting within several days or weeks after injury. Symptoms include headache, neck pain, dizziness, difficulty with memory and concentration, irritability, incoordination of fine motor control, generalized weakness, faintness, and others. An intracranial hematoma or epileptiform process should be ruled out. It is then important that the physician reassure his patient of the benign nature of this common syndrome. Psychiatric support and neuroleptic agents may be of benefit.

CONCLUSION

Over the past decade, there has been significant improvement in the mortality and morbidity of head trauma patients. This achievement has resulted from applying a few essential principles of head trauma management and an awareness of new developments in neurotrauma investigation. The most significant strides have resulted from (1) rapid transport of the patient and airway management, (2) early CT diagnosis and evacuation of mass lesions, and (3) intensive medical management including monitoring of cardiovascular status, ICP, and controlled ventilation. The authors have observed a marked reduction in patient morbidity and mortality over the past ten years attributed to an aggressive management of head injuries. More investigation and public education remains to be done to achieve further progress in treatment and prevention of head trauma.

REFERENCES

1. Allen SJ. Management of intracranial hypertension. In: Miner ME, Wagner KA (eds), Neurotrauma Treatment, Rehabilitation, and Related Issues. Boston, Butterworths, 1986, pp 41-54.
2. Andrews BT, Pitts LH, Lovely MP, et al. Is computed tomographic scanning necessary in patients with tentorial herniation? Results of immediate surgical exploration without computed tomography in 100 patients. Neurosurg, 1986, 19:408-414.
3. Becker DP, Miller JD, Ward JD, et al. The outcome from severe head injury with early diagnosis and intensive management. J Neurosurg, 1977, 47:491-502.
4. Bowers SA, Marshall LF. Outcome in 200 consecutive cases of severe head injury treated in San Diego County: A prospective analysis. Neurosurg, 1980, 6:237-242.
5. Boyd DR. Trauma — A controllable disease in 1980s. J Trauma, 1980, 20:14-24.

6. Bracken MB, Shepard MJ, Collins WF, et. al. A randomized controlled trial of methylpred-nisolone or naloxone in the treatment of acute spinal-cord injury. N Engl J Med, 1990, 322:1405-11.

7. Cairns CB, Fillipo D, Palladino GW, et al. Direct noninvasive assessment of brain metabolism during increased intracranial pressure: Potential therapeutic vistas. J Trauma, 1986, 26:863-868.

8. Clifton GL, Robertson CS, Grossman RG, et al. The metabolic response to severe head injury. J Neurosurg, 1984, 60:687-696.

9. Cooper PR. Delayed brain injury: Secondary insults. In: Becker DP, Povlishock JT (eds), Central Nervous System Trauma — Status Report. Washington, National Institutes of Health, 1985, pp 217-228.

10. Frankowski RF. The demography of head injury in the United States. In: Miner ME, Wagner KA (eds), Neurotrauma Treatment, Rehabilitation, and Related Issues. Boston, Butter-worths, 1986, pp 1-17.

11. Gennarelli TA, Spielman G, Longfitt TW, et al. The influence of the type of intracranial lesion on outcome from severe head injury: A multicenter study using a new classification system. J Neurosurg, 1982, 56:26-32.

12. Gennarelli TA, Thibault LE. Biomechanics of head injury. In: Wilkins RH, Rengachary SS (eds). Neurosurgery, Part III, Section A. New York, McGraw-Hill, 1985, pp 1531-1536.

13. Gentleman D, Jennett B. Hazards of inter-hospital transfer of comatose head injured patients. Lancet, 1981, 2:853-855.

14. Greenberg RP, Newlon PG, Hyatt MS, et al. Prognostic implications of early multimodality evoked potentials in severely head injured patients: A prospective study. J Neurosurg, 1981, 55:227-236.

15. Hadley MN, Grahm TW, Harrington T, et al. Nutritional support and neurotrauma: A critical review of early nutrition in forty-five acute head injury patients. Neurosurg, 1986, 19:367-373.

16. Hellams SE, Becker DP. Head injuries. Part 11: Lessons from a ten-year study. Virginia Med J, 1984, 111:206-211.

17. Jennett B, Bond M. Assessment of outcome after severe brain damage: A practical scale. Lancet, 1975, 1:480-484.

18. Jennett B, Teasdale G, Braackman R, et al. Predicting outcome in individual patients after severe head injury. Lancet, 1976, 1:1031-1034.

19. Jennett B, Teasdale G, Braakman R, et al. Prognosis of patients with severe head injury. Neurosurg, 1979, 4:283-289.

20. Jones TH, Morawetz RB, Crowell RM, et al. Threshold of focal cerebral ischemia in awake monkeys. J Neurosurg, 1981, 54:773-782.

21. Kalsbeek WD, Mclaurin RL, Harris BSH, et al. The National Head and Spinal Cord Injury Survey: Major Findings. J Neurosurg, 1980, 53 (Suppl):S19-S31.

22. Klauber MR, Toutant SM, Marshall LF. A model for predicting delayed intracranial hyper-tension following severe head injury. J Neurosurg, 1984, 61:695-699.

23. Kraus JF, Black MA, Hessol N. The incidence of acute brain injury and serious impairment in a defined population. Am J Epidemiol, 1984, 119:186-201.

24. Mackey-Hargadine J, Hall JW. Sensory evoked responses in head injury. J Am Paralysis Assoc, 1985, 2:187-206.

25. Marshall LF, Marshall SB. Medical management of intracranial pressure. In: Cooper PR (ed), Head Injury 2nd ed. Baltimore, Williams & Wilkins, 1987, pp 177-196.

26. Marshall LF, Toole BM, Bowers SA. The National Traumatic Coma Data Bank: Part II. Patients who talk and deteriorate: Implications for treatment. J Neurosurg, 1983, 59:285-288.

27. Marshall LF, Smith RW, Shapiro HM. The outcome with aggressive treatment in severe head injuries, Part 1: The significance of intracranial pressure monitoring. J Neurosurg, 1979, 50:20-25.

28. Miller JD. Prediction of outcome after head injury: A critical review. In: McLaurin RL (ed), Extracerebral Coollections. New York, Springer-Verlag, 1986, pp 229-247.
29. Miller JD, Becker DP, Ward JD, et al. Significance of intracranial hypertension in severe head injury. J Neurosurg, 1977, 47:503-516.
30. Miller JD, Sweet RC, Narayan R, et al. Early insults to the injured brain. JAMA, 1978, 240:439-442.
31. Muizelaar JP, Obrist WD. Cerebral blood flow and brain metabolism with brain injury. In: Becker DP, Povlishock JT (eds). Central Nervous System Trauma — Status Report. Washington, National Institutes of Health, 1985, pp 123-137.
32. Narayan RK, Kishore PRS, Becker DP, et al. Intracranial pressure: To monitor or not to monitor. J Neurosurg 1982, 56:650-659.
33. National Center for Health Statistics. Monthly Vital Statistics Report: Annual Report: Final Monthly Statistics, Vol 29, No 6, Suppl 2. Washington DC, US Government Printing Office, 1980:1-39 (DHHS Publication No PHS 80-1120), 1978.
34. National Center for Health Statistics. Advance report, final mortality statistics, 1980. Monthly vital statistics report, vol 32, no 4, Suppl. (DHHS Publication No PHS 83-1120). Hyattsville MD, Public Health Service, August 1983.
35. Obrist WD, Langfitt TW, Dolinskas CA, et al. Factors relating to intracranial hypertension in acute head injury. In: Ishii VS, Nagai H, Brook H (eds). Intracranial Pressure. Berlin-Heidelberg, Springer Verlag, 1983, pp 491-494.
36. Obrist WD, Langfitt TW, Jaggi JL, et al. Cerebral blood flow and metabolism in comatose patients with acute head injury. J Neurosurg, 1984, 61:241-253.
37. Overgaard J, Mosdale C, Tweed WA. Cerebral circulation after head injury, Part 3. Does reduced regional cerebral blood flow determine recovery of brain function after blunt head injury? J Neurosurg, 1981, 55:63-74.
38. Rose J, Valtonen S, Jennett B. Avoidable factors contributing to death after head injury. Br Med J, 1977, 2:615-618.
39. Saul TG, Ducker TB. Effects of intracranial pressure monitoring and aggressive treatment on mortality in severe head injury. J Neurosurg, 1982, 56:498-503.
40. Seelig JM, Becker DP, Miller JD, et al. Traumatic acute subdural hematoma: Major mortality reduction in comatose patients treated within four hours N Eng J Med, 1981, 304:1511-1518.
41. Stone JL, Lowe RJ, Jonasson O, et al. Acute subdural hematoma: direct admission to a trauma center yields improved results. J Trauma, 1986, 26:445-450.
42. Stone JL, Rifai MHS, Sugar O, et al. Subdural hematomas I — Acute subdural hematoma: Progress in definition, clinical pathology, and therapy. Surg Neurol, 1983, 19:216-231.
43. Stone JL. Nonsurgical management of increased intracranial pressure. Semin Neurol, 1989, 9:218-224.
44. Teasdale G, Jennett B. Assessment of coma and impaired consciousness. A practical scale. Lancet, 1974, 2:81-84.
45. Toutant SM, Klauber MR, Marshall LF, et al. Absent or compressed basal cisterns on first CT scan are ominous predictors of outcome in severe head injury. J Neurosurg, 1984, 61:691-694.
46. Van Dongen KJ, Braakman R. Late computed tomography in survivors of severe head injury. Neurosurg, 1980, 7:14-22.
47. Whitman S, Coonley-Hoganson R, Desai BT. Comparative head trauma experiences in two socioeconomically different Chicago-area communities: A population study. Am J Epidemiol, 1984, 119:570-580.

Chapter 2

Surgical Technique
in the Management of Head Injury

James L. Stone and Robert A. Moody

The following aspects of surgical therapy for head injury were presented in part at the Midwest Neuro-Trauma Seminar (AANS/CNS) given in Chicago in November, 1986. The surgical approaches outlined below have been used to advantage in the Cook County Hospital's Division of Neurosurgery over the past 15 years. These techniques evolved with the widespread diagnostic use of cerebral angiography in the 1960s and 1970s, and more liberal use of power instruments enabling the surgeon to rapidly perform a good-sized decompressive craniotomy bone flap. Also in the early to mid-1970s, the benefit of a large craniotomy for adequate clot removal and debridement of contusions and intracranial pressure (ICP) monitoring became better appreciated in selected patients. Our center cares for over 100 severe head injuries per year, the majority of which are secondary to blunt assaults or falls. Consequently we surgically treat many focal traumatic intracranial lesions such as subdural and extradural hematomas, cerebral contusions, and parenchymal cerebral hematomas. We hope these comments may benefit the neurosurgeon treating head injuries and acquaint the non-neurosurgeon with the clinical pathology encountered.

Acute Subdural Hematoma

Acute subdural hematoma (ASDH) is the most common traumatic intracranial hematoma requiring emergency surgery in the setting of severe head injury, with the highest morbidity and mortality. This lesion also serves as a paradigm for teaching the basic surgical approaches required to effectively handle complicated head injuries. Craniotomy is almost always required within 24 hours of injury to preserve life and function. Pupillary and brain stem findings are often present, with rapid clinical deterioration. The CT scan usually shows an extensive concave blood density collection with midline shift. Contusions and a variable amount of brain swelling are usually present. Early subacute subdural hematoma presenting 2 to 3 days after injury may require similar treatment.

We place a large sandbag under the shoulder, turn the head laterally 90°, ear in the center of horseshow headrest, to allow for a contralateral coronal ventriculostomy. The head is slightly elevated above the heart.

A generous skin incision, coronal or question mark, with the medial limb on the midline, and temporal extension to the zygomatic arch inferiorly is our standard approach. In all comatose patients, the temporal incision is opened first, and a craniectomy with partial clot removal precedes formal craniotomy. The temporalis muscle is removed with the cutting cautery and remains with the skin flap. A large (10 × 12 cm) fronto-temporo-parietal craniotomy is carried to the fronto-temporal skull base and within 1.5 to 2 cm of the midline. The basal exposure facilitates clot removal and hemostasis and it allows the involved hemisphere to move laterally away from the brain stem. Subfrontal or subtemporal clots may not show well on CT scan, but must not be missed. The dura is opened initially over the relatively silent basifrontal or anterior inferior temporal regions and based medially. After partial clot removal, the dural opening is carefully completed.

The subdural clot is irrigated from the cortical surface. Particularly adherent clot is often associated with the source of the hemorrhage – contused or lacerated cortical or dural vessels, bridging veins, or adhesion pedicles from old head injuries. Cerebral cortical contusions or lacerations may be continuous with intraparenchymal clot – usually temporal or frontal. Clot irrigation rapidly progresses in a circumferential fashion. The brain may be gently depressed with a large brain spatula as the saline irrigation stream is directed under the limits of dural exposure. Occasionally irrigation fluid will well up on the brain surface under the dura, in which case gentle depression of the brain surface away from the dura in several directions will release the trapped fluid. We back off from complete clot removal near the midline, lateral sinus, or poorly exposed regions. Although returning irrigation fluid will often be pink, any active bleeding must be stopped. Occasionally bridging veins to the superior sagittal sinus or the vein of Labbé must be controlled with silver clips.

We then reapproximate and begin to close the convexity dura as quickly as possible, since progressive intraoperative brain swelling is not uncommon with ASDH. A relaxing fascial graft or dural substitute is often required in the temporal and/or basifrontal regions, if swelling is marked. During dural closure one must avoid sharp dural kinks and edges by grafting the dura if necessary. Adequate dural closure prevents later cortical congestion and hemorrhagic infarction from the brain herniating around a dural or bone edge. When the brain is swollen at surgery and a large dural graft required, the bone flap is left out. About 10% of the time, the dura cannot be closed due to brain swelling after ASDH removal; gelfoam is placed about the edges and the scalp closed.

A contralateral ventriculostomy is preferred for ASDH, but any ICP monitor may be used. In cases of ASDH where anterior temporal or basifrontal contusion/laceration is prominent with a thinner or moderate sized subdural clot, basal areas are debrided first. When the brain is slacker and pulsates well, we gently pack the cavity with gelfoam and cottonoid and complete the dural opening and closure as above. A limited anterior temporal lobectomy is often required with ASDH (see below).

Anterior Temporal Lobe Parenchymal Hematoma/Contusion

These may present with primary or delayed onset. Patients may be obtunded or combative with or without focal signs such as muteness or hemiparesis. The CT scan often shows crowding or obliteration of basal cisterns with narrowing or shift of the third ventricle. The lateral ventricle may not be shifted unless contusion, edema, or middle cerebral ischemia extends posterosuperiorly. Sphenoidal contusion may involve the inferior frontal or temporal lobe diffusely.

The patient's head is positioned as for ASDH. A coronal incision is made at the zygoma 1 to 1.5 cm anterior to the external auditory meatus and extended vertically and gently forward. The scalp incision may curve posteriorly if a small or moderate extra-axial clot or significant posterior temporal contusion is present. A (3 × 3 cm) temporal craniectomy (or frontotemporal craniotomy) is performed to the base of the temporal fossa approaching the anterior tip. If mastoid cells are entered, they are obliterated by bone wax mixed with bacitracin powder. Following coagulation, the dura is opened over the anterior middle temporal gyrus. With the bovie sucker (lowered suction force) and bipolar cautery, soft, contused middle and inferior temporal gyri are removed posteriorly for about 3 to 4 cm from the tip. The most medial temporal white matter and the medial pial barrier are left undisturbed. Bipolar coagulation and gelfoam control the hemostasis. Adjacent devitalized brain tissue is also removed, being more conservative on the left side. With adequate decompression, the brain usually begins to pulsate well. A relaxing temporalis dural patch graft is almost always required due to dural shrinkage from coagulation. The dura may be tacked up to the deeper temporalis muscle fibers or bone edge.

At times, parenchymal cerebral hematoma/contusion can be located in the frontal or parietal lobe(s) and require surgical evacuation. Again the principles of adequate decompression and hemostasis, relaxing dural closure, and intensive postoperative monitoring apply. CT brain scans may have to be repeated often.

Acute or Subacute Epidural Hematoma

These usually appear on the CT scan as a biconvex blood density collection. They generally require a large craniotomy similar to ASDH, centered on the thicker areas of clot and in relation to vascular channels which may have been causative. In comatose patients, a partial localized craniectomy immediately precedes formal craniotomy. A lateral (park-bench) position for posterior fossa or parietal occipital hematomas near the midline is used. After epidural clot removal and extensive placement of tack-up sutures, the dura is opened if subdural lesions have been seen on CT scan. Drains are placed only if hemostasis is a problem. ICP is monitored postoperatively as in any severe head injury requiring surgery.

Chronic Subdural Hematoma

This entity is usually seen on CT scan as a hypodense extra-axial collection. Three burr holes are place in line with a possible craniotomy incision. On lateralized lesions, we try to turn the head (and shoulder) to avert postoperative frontal pneumocephalus. The initial burr hole is enlarged to observe for the extent (thickness) of subdural membrane formation, adequate fluid removal, and adequate visualization of the brain surface. We never hesitate to perform a craniotomy if any of the above problems are encountered, if loculation is suspected, or formed clot is present. We irrigate the brain surface with slightly warmed Lactated Ringer's solution. A drain (EVD type or small red rubber with extra holes) is only placed into a burr hole through which safe passage to the subdural space is easily accomplished so it irrigates freely. A closed drainage bag (or glove) is incorporated loosely into a full head dressing and after the first day placed on the bed adjacent to the patient. The drain is removed on the third day or sooner if it ceases to function or if CSF appears to be draining. The patient is kept flat for at least one day after the drain is removed.

Subdural Hygromas

Here we find clear or xanthochromic fluid in the absence of membrane formation. We place two burr holes to evacuate the often proteinaceous fluid, irrigate the brain surface, and place the subdural drain.

Depressed Skull Fracture

(Gunshot entrance or exit.) Generous simple scalp incisions, respecting major arterial supply to the scalp, are needed. We try to avoid stellate incisions over future skull defects and flap point ischemia. An adjacent burr hole for localization of the dural edge, followed by circumferential craniectomy and elevation of fragments follows next. In lateralized comminuted depressions within the temporalis muscle, we consider osteoplastic craniotomy. Hemorrhagic brain surface (or exposed tracts) and subcortical lesions must be adequately debrided. Depressed bone fragments to a depth of several centimeters should be removed if surrounded by non-viable brain, especially in non-eloquent cortical areas. A secure dural closure frequently requires a pericranium or fascial graft. If frontal air sinuses are encountered, they must be exenterated fully and obliterated with fat (anterior temporalis), muscle, or fascial bridge.

REFERENCES

1. Becker DP, Gade GF, Young HF, Feuerman PF. Diagnosis and treatment of head injury in adults. In: Youmans JR (ed), Neurological Surgery, ed 3, vol 3. Philadelphia, WB Saunders, 1989, pp 2017-2148.
2. Cooper PR. Post-traumatic intracranial mass lesions. In: Cooper PR (ed), Head Injury, ed 2. Baltimore, Williams & Wilkins, 1987, pp 238-284.
3. Stone JL, Rifai MSH, Sugar O, Lang RGR, Oldershaw JB, Moody RA. Subdural hematomas: I. Acute subdural hematoma: Progress in definition, clinical pathology, and therapy. Surg Neurol, 1983, 19:216-231.

Chapter 3
=========

Pediatric Head Injuries:
Mechanisms, Management, and Sequelae

George R. Cybulski and James L. Stone

An approach to understanding the mechanisms, management, and sequelae of pediatric head injury must include recognition of age dependent variability that exists within the pediatric population. For example, the treatment plan as well as pathogenetic considerations differ widely between the newborn infant with a frontal lobe contusion/hematoma (Figure 3.1) and an adolescent with a similar-appearing traumatic condition. This age-dependent variability is a function of unique characteristics of the developing brain and its encasing structures. Therefore, clinical and pathologic consequences of head injury will vary over time as age dependent changes occur in the nervous elements and their coverings.

HEAD INJURY IN THE NEWBORN

While the immature skull with its open sutures and fontanelles allows for molding of the head to pass through the birth canal, this adaptive function also exposes the underlying brain to unique forms of injury.

Head trauma in the newborn is predominantly related to obstetrical causes [14,16,22]. Although this incidence is diminishing because of improved techniques, it still continues to be the cause of approximately 2% of all neonatal mortality [14,16]. The main types of perinatal head trauma include extracranial hemorrhage, skull fracture, and intracranial hemorrhage/contusion [14,22,29].

29

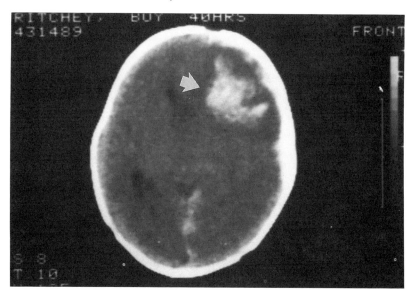

Figure 3.1. CT scan of newborn infant. Prolonged labor, forceps delivery. Frontal (arrow) and interhemispheric contusional hemorrhage treated conservatively, with resolution.

EXTRACRANIAL HEMORRHAGE IN THE NEWBORN

The forms of neonatal extracranial hemorrhage are classified according to the different tissue planes of scalp in which they occur: caput succedaneum is hemorrhagic edema into the skin ad superficial fascia, subaponeurotic or subgaleal hemorrhage occurs between the epicranial aponeurosis and the periosteum, and cephalhematoma is the designation for bleeding beneath the periosteum over the outer skull surface (Figure 3.2). The incidence of these predominant forms of perinatal extracranial hemorrhage is not known but they are not uncommon..

Caput succedaneum, an edematous swelling of the presenting scalp of the infant's head, is thought to be due to circulatory stasis from compression exerted by the uterine-cervical ring during vaginal delivery. It is a circumscribed lesion that is "boggy" with pitting edema. It usually resolves in a few days without treatment.

While caput succedaneum is a localized process, subgaleal or subaponeurotic hemorrhage occurs within a widespread potential space, and thus can become a significant hemorrhage. These forms of extracranial hemorrhage are usually caused by torsional or shearing forces that rupture deeper scalp vessels. The key to recognition is observation of an enlarging process beneath the scalp. Skull fracture with dural tear and cerebrospinal fluid accumulation must be excluded. Treatment of subgaleal hemorrhage includes monitoring for the effects of blood loss, hyperbilirubinemia, and coagulopathy. Some authors have advocated aseptic aspiration followed by compressive head wrapping. However, conservative management is usually appropriate and effective [16,28].

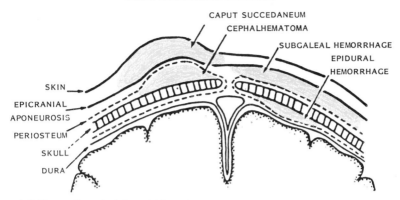

Figure 3.2. Traumatic perinatal cranial hematomas.

Cephalhematoma is a general term that can refer to any form of scalp hematoma. However, in the context of neonatal head trauma, cephalhematoma is used to denote subperiosteal bleeding. This type of hemorrhage is self-limited by periosteal attachments and does not cross suture lines. Formerly, when mid-forceps deliveries were common in obstetric practice, the incidence of this type of hemorrhage was higher than the 1% to 2% of today [16]. The parietal bones are most often affected via a mechanism thought to involve shearing or torsional forces that elevate periosteum from bone. The sudden release of pressure on scalp vessels after vaginal delivery may be an additional mechanical factor leading to cephalhematoma formation. Monitoring for blood loss by hematocrit determination and observation of the infant's spontaneity, tonus, and respiratory status is usually the only treatment required for this variety of neonatal hemorrhage.

SKULL FRACTURES IN THE NEWBORN

Generally, the poorly mineralized newborn skull with its membranous sutures allows extensive compression and distortion with minimal risk of fracture. However, a form of depressed skull fracture termed a "ping-pong" fracture (Figure 3.3) occurs with enough regularity to be discussed. The pathogenesis is thought to be impaction against the sacral promontory during labor [1] or secondary to the application of forceps during delivery [14,16]. If the depression occurs in an area that is not cosmetically significant, such as the parietal region (Figure 3.4), or if there is no overriding of bone edges, then nonsurgical management may supervene as brain growth and skull re-modeling will usually occur and reduce the fracture [19].

Linear fractures most commonly occur in the parietal bones during complicated deliveries, especially involving forceps or feto-pelvic disproportion. The fracture may be associated with any form of extracranial hemorrhage previously discussed or, in rare instances, an epidural hematoma. The fracture itself is usually not of clinical significance but serves as a warning for further intracranial injury. Skull x-ray must be repeated several months later to rule out a growing skull fracture (leptomeningeal

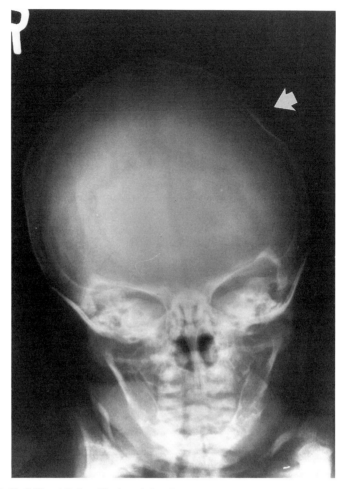

Figure 3.3. Skull film, AP view. Newborn infant forceps delivery. Ping-pong fracture (arrow).

cyst) [3]. The occurrence of growing skull fractures after linear but often diastatic skull fractures develop more commonly before the age of 3 years [24]. Surgical correction of the dural defect is necessary.

Occipital osteodiastasis is a rare traumatic separation of squamous and lateral portions of the occipital bone that most commonly occurs during breech delivery [22,29]. The head of the fetus is trapped beneath the symphysis pubis causing inward suboccipital hinging and pressure. With more severe injury, adjacent occipital sinuses are torn by the displaced lateral portions of the occipital bone, causing posterior fossa subdural hematoma, cerebellar hemorrhage, and laceration. This type of severe lesion may be rapidly fatal, and prior to computed tomographic (CT) brain scanning, was principally diagnosed at autopsy. Hydrocephalus may be detected and treated in less serious posterior fossa hematomas.

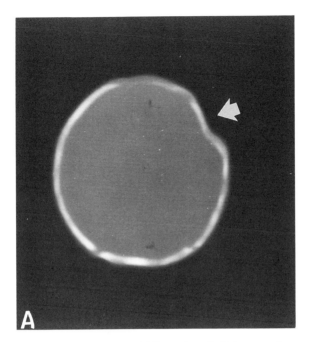

Figure 3.4A. CT scan, same case as Figure 3.3. Elevated surgically because of cosmetic deformity.

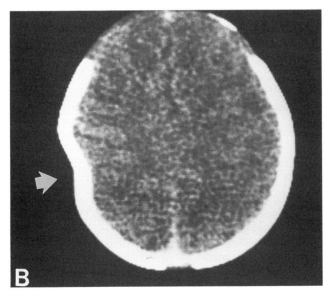

Figure 3.4B. CT scan of newborn infant. Temporoparietal ping-pong fracture treated conservatively, with resolution.

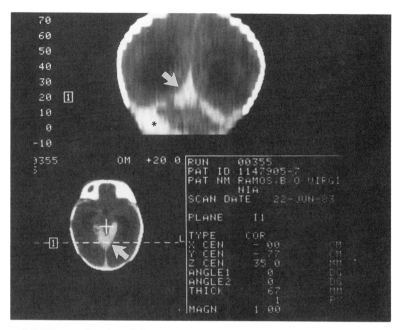

Figure 3.5. CT scan of newborn infant at two days of age. Falcotentorial hemorrhage (arrow), posterior fossa subdural hematoma (asterisk), and hydrocephalus. Recovery following emergency surgical decompression of the posterior fossa and ventriculoperitoneal shunting two weeks later.

CT scanning and trans-fontanelle ultrasound of the brain via the anterior fontanelle (Figure 3.5) have more recently established the diagnosis of posterior fossa subdural hematoma at a stage when evacuation of the hematoma may be performed successfully [26]. Any infant with a complicated delivery who exhibits signs of increased intracranial pressure (ICP), such as bulging fontanelle, suture separation, bradycardia or apneic episodes should be suspected of having this disorder.

INTRACRANIAL HEMORRHAGE IN THE NEWBORN

Hemorrhage into the subdural space can occur secondary to falcotentorial laceration or rupture of any of the other major venous sinuses or superficial cerebral veins during delivery[29]. This occurs as a result of forces of labor leading to crushing, shearing, or torsional actions associated with extreme skull molding. Diagnosis depends upon suspicion of increased intracranial pressure and CT scanning or ultrasonography to image the lesion. Hemorrhages may be supra or infratentorial in location. Therapy depends on the degree of mass effect caused by lesion. Fluid collections may be evacuated with burr hole drainage, but solid clots require a larger craniotomy.

Cerebral contusion often occurs simultaneously with subdural hematomas. Contusions usually can be managed conservatively when the thickness of the subdural hematoma measures less than 5 mm on the CT scan and is not causing mass effect.

HEAD INJURY DURING FIRST 2 YEARS OF LIFE

Epidemiology

Although head injury is a major cause of disability and mortality in children, the epidemiology of such injuries, especially in the first 2 years, is not well described [2]. This difficulty is due in part to the fact that the usual sources of data on such incidence (death certificates, hospital admission diagnoses, emergency room diagnoses, and surveys) probably represent only a small portion of the actual total of pediatric head injuries [2]. The task is further complicated when concepts and definitions derived from experience with head injury in the adult population are used for the pediatric age group. However, a few studies provide useful information to differentiate the particulars of pediatric head injuries from that of adults [2,13].

It has been reported that in injuries for which medical care is sought in children — the head is most frequently involved [13,18]. This is particularly true for the preschool age group. According to a review of various hospital admission diagnoses, the percentage of children under 2 years of age who were admitted to a hospital for head injury ranged from 5.5% to 25% [13]. In children under two years of age, the main causes of head injury are falls, child abuse, and motor vehicle accidents [13,15].

Falls can be grouped into two categories: (1) falls — from cribs, cots, dressing tables, or high chairs — occurring early in life and (2) falls due to attempts at ambulation that occur as the child approaches two years of age. Failure of parental attention and supervision is the major contributing factor to both types of falls. In urban areas, falls from windows are a leading cause of death in children less that 5 years of age, with a peak incidence around age 2 [13,15].

Motor vehicle accidents account for the highest percentage of death and injury among infants under 6 months (9 per 100,000) [13]. This has been attributed to the malleable condition of the infant's skull during this time period and to the greater chance of the infant being in the front seat or held in the arms of a passenger who would then act to crush the infant between his body and the dashboard in the event of an accident. The use of infant restraint systems goes a long way toward preventing these injuries.

Child abuse is considered the predominant source of nonaccidental head trauma in children less than 2 years of age [13,18]. As opposed to the approximately 1% incidence of skull fractures in infants accidentally falling from cribs or furniture, abused infants are more likely to suffer skull fractures (Figure 3.6). It has been observed that 29% of skull fractures in infants less than 18 months of age were the result of child abuse [13]. The characteristics of the skull fracture may arouse

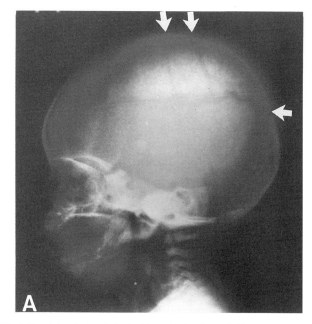

Figure 3.6A. Skull film, lateral view. Infant with multiple, diastatic linear skull fractures (arrows), known to have been abused and shaken. Survival with intellectual disturbance.

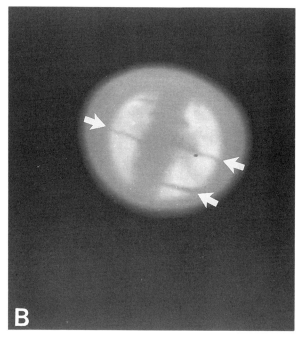

Figure 3.6B. CT scan bone windows, same case as Figure 3.6A.

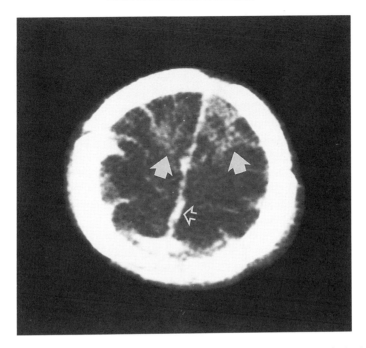

Figure 3.7. CT scan. Same case as Figure 3.6. Subarachnoid (arrows) and interhemispheric hemorrhage (open arrow).

suspicion of abuse, especially when the fracture is comminuted rather than linear. Evidence of other injuries or fractures elsewhere may also indicate child abuse.

In addition to direct trauma to the infant's skull resulting in fracture, another form of child abuse with head injury is called the whiplash-shaken infant syndrome [10]. As suggested by the name, the infant is shaken by the extremities with whiplash of the head, causing shearing forces to bridging vessels and resultant subdural, subarachnoid, and subpial hemorrhage (Figure 3.7). Head injury from abuse can also take on the appearance of the broad spectrum of cerebral injury, including cerebral contusion, compound comminuted skull fractures, and subdural hematoma [20].

Mechanism

The unique age-dependent variability of pediatric head injury is most apparent in consideration of the pathogenetic mechanisms in the age category of infant to 2 years [24].

Courville described some of these features from autopsy studies in which he reported a relative infrequency of contrecoup lesions during infancy [11]. This is in contrast to an 85% to 95% frequency of contrecoup injury in the adult patient. Courville found that contrecoup injury increases between infancy and age 3 and then levels off to adult percentages.

Another unique finding with blunt head trauma in infants less than 5 months of age is that of cerebral white matter tears. These tears occur parallel to the surface of the brain in contrast to cortical contusion that occurs in more mature brains [13,30].

Postulated mechanisms behind these patterns include the theory that the plastic nature of the skull during this time period allows for less movement of the brain without impaction against the skull (contrecoup phenomena) and the friability of the poorly myelinated cerebrum (white matter tears) [13,21].

Unfortunately, the presence of these structural modifying factors, while producing a unique pattern of damage from head injury in the infant population, does not offer a mitigating effect. Rather, younger children suffer greater damage than their older counterparts from deceleration-impact injuries in falls and from acceleration-burst injuries due to blows such as occur with child abuse [13].

Raimondi and others have observed that the separation between good and bad outcome from head injury in childhood is closely correlated with the time of closure of the anterior fontanelle [13]. A higher incidence of skull fracture is clearly evident in open-fontanelle group of children — generally less than 1 year of age before the anterior fontanelle is completely closed [13]. Along with the higher incidence of skull fracture in the open-fontanelle/under age 2 group is a concomitant risk of cerebral damage and documented greater morbidity and mortality rates [8,13,24].

Management

Because a small number of children with seemingly minor head injuries develop potentially lethal complications such as an epidural hematoma (Figure 3.8), special attention and vigilance are the key factors in management. Consequently, in our evaluation and treatment of head injury in the pediatric age group, we tend to avoid labels such as a minor or moderate head injury which may tend to give a false sense of confidence. Rather, we stress concentration on early thorough evaluation and serial observation.

The Glasgow Coma Score (GCS) is a standardized method of evaluating the degree of severity of head injury in adults. However, it is not readily applicable to infants or toddlers because of the obvious reliance on varying degrees of higher integrative function (e.g., obeying commands, being oriented) [23]. A normal infant would not score better than 2 of a possible 5 on the verbal exam of the Glasgow Coma Score.

Therefore, we use a modified form of evaluation, the Infant Coma Score (ICS) (Table 3.1) which has three categories of assessment and a 15 point total as does the Glasgow Coma Score. This Infant Coma Score utilizes best responses to auditory-visual stimuli, nature of the cry, and consolability of the baby.

Any infant or toddler who is brought to our emergency department with a history of head injury is initially evaluated for the basic ABCs (airway, breathing, circulation)

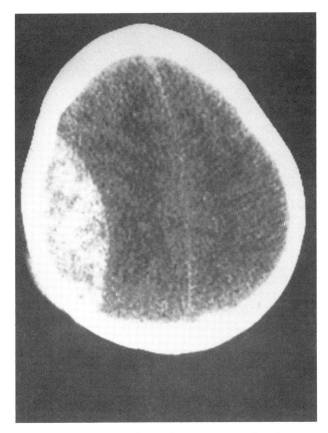

Figure 3.8. CT scan showing a temporoparietal epidural hematoma. Complete recovery following timely removal of the clot.

of resuscitation. Shock is generally not attributed to head injury, with the exception of the infant with a large intracranial hematoma.

A rapid but complete physical examination is performed including head circumference and neurological examination for staging by the Infant Coma Scale. This provides the baseline score against which serial exams are to be compared. Portable x-rays including lateral, antero-posterior, and Towne views are performed in the emergency room. Ultrasound may be performed through an open fontanelle.

CT brain scanning is obtained if skull films reveal a prominent fracture or diastasis, Infant Coma Score is 13 or less, focal neurologic findings are present on examination, persistent vomiting or if there is an open or penetrating skull injury. Intubation prior to transport to CT is indicated for patients with ICS scores of 7 or less.

Seizure prophylaxis is given with Dilantin (phenytoin) — loading dose of 10 to 15 mg/kg no faster than 50 mg/minute, and 5 mg/kg per day maintenance. Dilantin is given by intravenous injection when brain tissue is apparent on physical examination,

Table 3.1. Infant Coma Scale

	Eyes
4	Spontaneous
3	To speech
2	To pain
1	No response
	Best Motor
6	Spontaneous
5	Localizes pain
4	Withdraws to pain
3	Flexion to pain decorticate
2	Extension to pain decerebrate
1	No response
	(Use only one category of the following two)
	Age > 2 years: Best Verbal Response
5	Oriented
4	Confused
3	Inappropriate
2	Incomprehensible
1	No response
	Age < 2 years: Best response to Auditory/Visual Stimulus
5	Social, follows objects
4	Cries, consolable
3	Persistent cry, lethargy
2	Agitated/restless
1	No response
	Score
15	Normal
13-14	Mildly abnormal
9-12	Moderately abnormal
3- 8	Severely abnormal

with CT evidence of intracranial hemorrhage, cerebral laceration or contusion, or prior history of seizure disorder.

CT scanning is the definitive diagnostic test and if positive for a depressed skull fracture, epidural or subdural hematoma, or intracerebral hematoma with mass effect, then the appropriate neurosurgical decompressive measures are undertaken.

Comatose children without surgically significant lesions on CT brain scan have an intracranial pressure monitor placed (subarachnoid bolt, Camino parenchymal or intraventricular catheter) for intracranial pressure readings. Normal ICP ranges from 1.5 to 5.9 mmHg for infants and 3 to 7 mmHg for children [6,7,12].

The goal in treating pediatric head injury is to maintain ICP below 16 to 18 mmHg. When ICP is elevated, the basic strategy to lower ICP consists of hyperventilation to a $PaCO_2$ of 22 to 25 mmHg, elevation of the head 25° to 30° with good midline positioning to avoid kinking of the jugular veins, and diuretics (mannitol up to 1 gm/kg and low doses of Lasix) for dehydration of the brain. Ventricular drainage, in certain cases, may be beneficial.

Children in coma who do not demonstrate diffuse cerebral edema on CT scan usually can have their intracranial pressure controlled with these measures [7,12,13]. However, another group of children exhibit diffuse cerebral swelling with raised ICP that may not respond to these conventional techniques [6]. Barbiturate therapy is an alternative in this group [7,12,13]. Barbiturates are known to have effects upon reducing ICP on the basis of their vasoconstrictive action, scavenging of free radicals, and reduction of cerebral metabolic requirements. Pentobarbital, a short-acting barbiturate, is usually given in a 3 to 5 mg/kg loading dose, with 0.5 to 0.3 mg/kg/hr as maintenance for a blood level of 35 to 50 mg/ml. EEG burst-suppression and/or control of ICP serves as a guide for maximum therapy. The cerebral perfusion pressure (CPP, or mean arterial pressure – MAP – minus ICP) must be maintained at greater than 50 to 60 mmHg using vasopressors if needed.

HEAD INJURY IN OLDER CHILDREN

After 2 years of age, the skull and brain more closely approximate that of the adult; however, the types of cerebral injury observed in children indicate that the maturing brain still maintains a different age-dependent variability of response to trauma. For example, traumatic intracerebral hematomas occur 3 times more often in adults than in children; and acute subdural hematomas occur in children only about 25% as often as in adults [2,23,24]. In addition, cerebral contusions are less common in children (16%) than in adults (33%) [30].

Conversely, diffuse axonal shearing injuries more commonly occur in pediatric head injury than is seen in adults [21,30]. The pathogenetic mechanism behind shearing injuries was originally described in children involved in high speed motor vehicle accidents [27]. Children with this injury often present to the hospital in a decerebrate state with deep coma. On CT scan, ventricles are usually small; and deep hemispheric, diencephalic, or midbrain contusional hemorrhages may be found (Figure 3.9). The smaller intraparenchymal hematomas associated with shearing injuries in children in general do not require surgical evacuation (Figure 3.10) [24]. Management of head injury in older children follows the same principles already described for the younger age group; that is, surgically amenable lesions such as compound depressed skull fractures or epidural or subdural hematomas are corrected and ICP is monitored and treated according to the previously described protocol.

OUTCOME OF PEDIATRIC HEAD INJURY

Outcome and sequelae of pediatric head injury follows the general pattern that "the younger the child, the greater the damage to the brain from blunt head trauma"

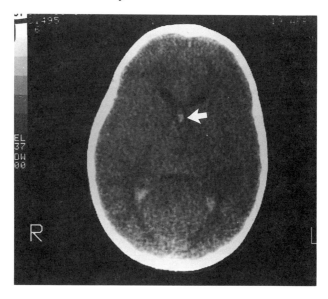

Figure 3.9. CT scan of a 15 year old girl injured in a high speed vehicular accident. Anterior callosal (arrow) and intraventricular hemorrhage. The patient remained in a chronic vegetative state despite intensive medical treatment including intracranial pressure monitoring.

[23]. It has been observed that 13.4% of children less than 12 months of age have a poor outcome after blunt head trauma, compared to a 4.9% poor outcome in the age group of 1 to 3 years (Figure 3.11) [23].

However, problems occur in attempting to derive a composite outcome for the complete age ranges seen in pediatric head injury because of the small sample size when compared with the large numbers of adult head injuries. Large pediatric referral centers such as Children's Hospital in Philadelphia report an encouraging 5% mortality rate for children with Glasgow Coma Scores of less than 8 [5], and other centers with aggressive treatment protocols for ICP management report 14% to 16% mortality rates [25]. Studies with mortality rates of 33% to 40% question the effects that differences in pattern of referral and triage may have upon outcome statistics [4,17].

By anatomical lesion, the following pediatric head injury rates occur: In the pre-CT scan era, mortality from epidural hematoma ranged from 26% to 30% [5]. With rapid transport to a trauma center and prompt CT scanning, early recognition and treatment has decreased these figures dramatically, approaching zero in a number of institutions [5]. Acute subdural hematomas are likewise recognized earlier with the CT scan; but fortunately this is a relatively rare lesion (approximately 5%) in children, with a dismal 85% mortality in one operative series of children [24]. However, it appears that the mortality for children 20 years and younger is less after severe head injury than the comparable mortality in the adult population, and the degree of primary irreversible brain injury sustained by children is frequently less

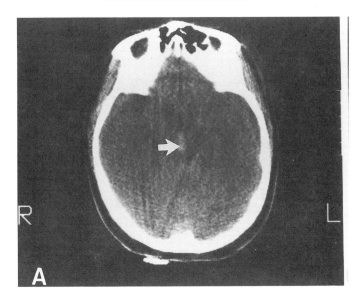

Figure 3.10A. CT brain scan of the same patient as Figure 3.9. Midbrain hemorrhage (arrow).

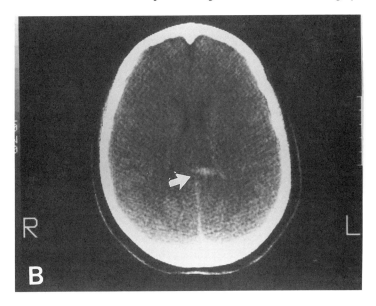

Figure 3.10B. CT brain scan of the same patient as Figure 3.9. Hemorrhage in the posterior corpus callosum (arrow).

than in adults [4]. Therefore, attention to mitigating secondary injuries (i.e., anoxia, hypercarbia, delayed treatment) is as paramount in the pediatric as in the adult age group.

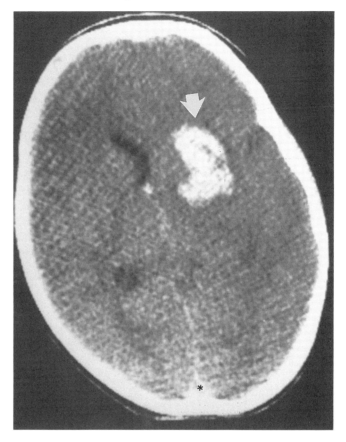

Figure 3.11. CT brain scan, 3 year old struck by automobile. Deep frontal hemorrhage (arrow) and posterior interhemispheric hemorrhage (asterisk). Conservative treatment with intracranial pressure monitoring. Excellent recovery from a comatose state.

RECOVERY AND SEQUELAE

Severe neurological dysfunction upon admission does not prevent a satisfactory recovery in children and adolescents. The majority of children (over than 90%) under age 15 who survive a severe craniocerebral injury are able to recover beyond a chronic vegetative or severely disabled state [24]. In a study of 344 patients under age 18 who had severe closed-head injuries and were comatose for over 24 hours, 73% regained independence in ambulation and self-care [9]. The degree of recovery was closely correlated with duration of coma. Coma lasting 24 hours or less without CT evidence of focal damage is rarely associated with permanent neuropsychological sequelae, whereas coma of more than 3 days' duration is associated with a drop in intelligence quotient. However, coma of less than 6 weeks is still associated with a return to independent function in over 90% of children [27].

Compared with similarly managed adults, children are more apt to experience seizures at each level of injury severity. However, early seizures may not lead to post-traumatic epilepsy. In fact, it has been shown that the frequency of late epilepsy is less for children than for adults [5,24].

CONCLUSION

The successful control of many pediatric infectious diseases has brought trauma to the forefront as the predominant cause of mortality in children. Although it cannot be precisely determined, head injury figures prominently as a source of mortality and morbidity in the pediatric age group.

Head injury in children is a unique entity whose assessment and management must be separated from that of adult patients. It is recognized that within the pediatric population, age-dependent variability of injury mechanisms and pathology is based upon unique characteristics of the maturing nervous system and its coverings. Recognition of these concepts will allow an appropriate treatment plan for each child — which should further improve the outcome from head injury.

REFERENCES

1. Alexander E Jr, David CH Jr. Intra-uterine fracture of the infant's skull. J Neurosurg, 1969, 30:446-454.
2. Annegers JF. The epidemiology of head trauma in children. In: Shapiro K (ed), Pediatric Head Trauma. New York Futura Publishing, 1983, pp 1-10.
3. Arseni C, Ciurea AV. Clinicotherapeutic aspects in the growing skull fracture: A review of the literature. Child's Brain. 1981, 8:161-172.
4. Berger MS, Pitts LH, Lovely M, Edwards MSB, Bartkowski HM. Outcome from severe head injury in children and adolescents. J Neurosurg, 1985, 62:194-199.
5. Bruce DA, Shut L, Bruno LA, Wood JH, Sutton LN. Outcome following severe head injuries in children. J Neurosurg, 1978, 48:679-688.
6. Bruce DA, Abass A, Bilaniuk L, Dolinskas C, Obrist W, Uzzell B. Diffuse cerebral swelling following head injuries in children: The syndrome of "Malignant brain edema". J Neurosurg 1981, 54:170-178.
7. Bruce DA. Clinical care of the severely head injured child. In: Shapiro K (ed), Pediatric Head Trauma. New York, Futura Publishing, 1983, pp 27-44.
8. Bruce DA. Outcome following head trauma in childhood. In: Shapiro K (ed), Pediatric Head Trauma. New York, Futura Publishing, 1983, pp 213-222.
9. Brink JD, Imbus C, Woo-Sam J. Physical recovery after severe closed head trauma in children and adolescents. J Pediatrics. 1980, 97:721-727.
10. Caffey J. The whiplash shaken infant syndrome: Manual shaking by the extremities with whiplash-induced intracranial and intraocular bleedings, linked with residual permanent brain damage and mental retardation. Pediatrics, 1974, 54:396-403.
11. Courville CB. Contrecoup injuries of the brain in infancy: Remarks on the mechanism of fatal traumatic lesions of early life. Arch Surg, 1965, 90:157-165.
12. Dennis GC, Stein F. The management of increased intracranial pressure in children. J Nat Med Assoc, 1983, 75:1189-1196.

13. DiRocco C. Velardi F. Epidemiology and etiology of craniocerebral trauma in the first two years of life. In: Raimondi AJ, Choux M, DiRocco C (eds), Head Injuries in the Newborn and Infant. New York Springer-Verlag, 1986, pp 125-139.
14. Gresham EL. Birth trauma. Pediatr Clin North Am, 1975, 22:317-328.
15. Hall JR, Reyes HM, Horvat M, Meller JL, Stein R. The mortality of childhood falls. J Trauma, 1989, 29:1273-1275.
16. Hovind KH. Traumatic birth injuries. In: Raimondi AJ, Choux M, DiRocco C (eds), Head Injuries in the Newborn and Infant. New York Springer-Verlag, 1986, pp 88-109.
17. Humphreys RP, Jaimovich R, Hendrick EB, Hoffman HJ. Outcome of severe head injury in children: Is 6% mortality realistic? (Abstr). Can J Neurol Sci, 1983, 10:139.
18. Jamison DL, Kaye HH. Accidental head injury in childhood. Arch Dis Child, 1974, 49:376-381.
19. Loeser JD, Kilburn HL, Jolley T. Management of depressed skull fracture in the newborn. J Neurosurg, 1976, 44:62-64.
20. McClelland CQ, Rekate H, Kaufman B, Persse L. Cerebral injury in child abuse: A changing profile. Child's Brain, 1980, 7:225-235.
21. McLaurin RJ, Towbin R. Cerebral damage. In: Raimondi AJ, Choux M, DiRocco C (eds), Head Injuries in the Newborn and Infant. New York Springer-Verlag, 1986, pp 183-201.
22. Pape KE, Wigglesworth JS. Haemorrhage, Ischaemia and the Perinatal Brain. London, William Heinemann Medical Books, 1979, pp 66-71.
23. Raimondi AJ, Hirschauer J. Clinical criteria – children's coma score and outcome scale – For decision making in managing head-injured infants and toddlers. In: Raimondi AJ, Choux M, DiRocco C (eds), Head Injuries in the Newborn and Infant. New York Springer-Verlag, 1986, pp 141-150.
24. Shapiro K. Special considerations for the pediatric age group. In: Cooper PR (ed), Head Injury 2nd ed. Baltimore MD, Williams and Wilkins, 1987, pp 367-389.
25. Shapiro K, Marmarou A. Mechanism and treatment of intracranial hypertension in the head injured child. In: Shapiro K (ed), Pediatric Head Trauma. New York, Futura Publishing, 1983, pp 45-67.
26. Stone JL. Posterior fossa subdural hematomas in newborns. J Neurosurg, 1985, 62:626.
27. Stover SL, Zeiger HE Jr. Head injury in children and teenagers: Functional recovery correlated with duration of coma. Arch Phys Med Rehab, 1976, 57:201-205.
28. Strich SJ. Shearing of nerve fibres as a cause of brain damage due to head injury. Lancet, 1961, 2:443-448.
29. Volpe JJ. Neurology of the Newborn. Philadelphia, WB Saunders, 1981, pp 239-261.
30. Zimmerman RA, Bilaniuk LT. Radiology of pediatric craniocerebral trauma. In: Shapiro K (ed), Pediatric Head Trauma. New York, Futura Publishing, 1983, pp 69-142.
31. Zimmerman RA, Bilaniuk LT, Genneralli T. Computed tomography of shearing injuries of the cerebral white matter. Radiology, 1978, 127:393-396.

Chapter 4

Cerebral Blood Flow and Metabolism After Severe Head Injury

J. Paul Muizelaar and Walter D. Obrist

INTRODUCTION

There are many techniques for measuring cerebral blood flow (CBF) in vivo and all have been used with traumatic brain injury: the classic Kety Schmidt method using nitrous oxide [24]; wash-out of gamma-ray-emitting radioactive tracers, mainly [133]xenon but occasionally [85]krypton [38], either injected into one of the carotid arteries [10,13,21,22,23,37,79,80,81], administered by inhalation [69], or injected intravenously [9,11,75,76,100]; wash-out or wash-in of stable xenon monitored with repeated computerized tomographic (CT) scanning [106]; transit time of rapidly intravenously injected radiographic dye monitored with very fast serial CT scanning [107]; Doppler flow velocity measurements with probes inserted around one or both internal carotid arteries in the neck [27]; and ocular pneumoplethysmography [26]. Positron emission tomography (PET) scanning is also well suited to measure CBF, but apparently it is too cumbersome to use in the acute state of severe head injury. PET scanning has recently been used for glucose metabolism measurements in the more chronic stages of head injury [49]. We are presently investigating the possible use of thermodilution CBF measurements with a probe left on the cortical surface after surgery for subdural or traumatic intracerebral hematomas. Other techniques such as CBF measurement with magnetic resonance imaging (MRI) scanning are being investigated in other laboratories. Thus there are at least eight different

47

techniques in existence for measuring CBF after human head injury and others are being scrutinized. Yet, many questions relating to CBF and metabolism with traumatic brain injury remain unanswered. In this chapter we will define some of the questions which are to be addressed with CBF measurements, present our own data and discuss the literature relevant to those questions, and speculate on future developments. Moreover, form and function of the cerebral circulation as it relates to severe head injury are discussed. Parts of these general considerations have been discussed on earlier occasions [48,70].

NORMAL CEREBRAL CIRCULATION AS IT RELATES TO TRAUMA

The intracranial arteries and their branches can be arbitrarily divided into a conduction system, a resistance system, and an exchange system.

The *conduction system* is formed by the large and medium sized arteries. They can be made angiographically visible so that their diameter may be assessed in vivo. Despite the name conduction system, the larger arteries and surface vessels of the brain account for a greater portion of vascular resistance than is found in other vascular beds. Thus, the fall in pressure from the extracranial internal carotid artery to the larger pial arteries is equal to 39% to 51% [19,34,42,94,98,99] or, assuming that inflow pressure at capillary level is still 30 mmHg, conductive vessels contribute 60% to 70% of precapillary vascular resistance. This stems from the fact that the large cerebral arterial branches have long lengths and cerebral arterioles have comparatively much shorter lengths [25].

The *resistance system* is formed by the arterioles, metarterioles, and small thoroughfare channels. The arterioles have a very important function in cerebral autoregulation, as they can rapidly dilate or constrict [42]. The metarterioles and thoroughfare channels contain precapillary sphincters responsible for regulating the flow of blood to the capillary bed. Vasomotion is a physiological property of the microcirculation [109]. It is a regularly occurring series of partial constrictions and relaxations of metarterioles and precapillary sphincters at intervals of 30 seconds to several minutes. The result is a waxing and waning of flow through the capillary bed. At any given time, flow may be present in one portion of the capillary bed and absent in an adjacent portion because the precapillary sphincters are closed. This alternating constriction and relaxation of precapillary sphincters produces complex hemodynamic changes in the microcirculation. Although most observations of vasomotion have been in structures such as the ear and the mesentery of experimental animals, vasomotion is also a property of the microcirculation of the brain [90].

The *exchange* of gases, nutrition, and metabolites takes place mainly in the capillaries. Although capillaries are very numerous, especially in the gray matter, they still present a fair amount of resistance to flow, mainly because in humans, their diameter of 6 μ is slightly smaller than that of an erythrocyte [14]. This fact is important because it implies that erythrocytes must be deformed in order to pass through the capillaries. Changes in erythrocyte deformability, such as can be induced by the administration of mannitol [12], can lead to appreciable changes in resistance to flow in the capillary bed.

AUTOREGULATION

There are several ways of defining autoregulation. Taking CBF as a starting point, one definition could read: Increase of CBF with higher metabolic demands of the brain and decrease of CBF with lower demands (metabolic autoregulation) and constant CBF despite decrease or increase of perfusion pressure (pressure autoregulation).

Another definition is based upon vessel diameter changes: Dilation of resistance vessels with higher metabolic demands of the brain or with imminent lower supply of nutrients — mainly oxygen, or, conversely, vasoconstriction occurring in response to lower cerebral demands or higher supply. This definition contains the two classic arms of autoregulation, i.e., metabolic autoregulation and pressure regulation. However, blood viscosity autoregulation which we recently described [71,72], can also be included.

Metabolic autoregulation involves changes in vascular diameter produced by alteration in the demands of the cerebral tissue for oxygen and glucose. Normally there is a tight coupling between the demands of cerebral tissue for O_2 and glucose, and the volume of blood flowing through that tissue; although for a number of years, it was believed that the blood flow to the brain was stable under all conditions of activity. Measurements of CBF during a wide spectrum of activity — ranging from intense mental activity, exercise, apprehension, to sleep — disclosed a remarkably stable level of blood flow [40,58,92,96]. Only extreme changes in activity such as those occurring during seizures, coma, or hypothermia revealed appreciable changes in cerebral blood flow [7,53]. However, these extreme circumstances produce side effects, such as blood pressure changes, which can make the changes in cerebral blood flow hard to appreciate. The introduction of techniques for measurements of regional cerebral blood flow in localized area revealed and close relationship between regional cerebral blood flow and the activity of areas of the cerebral cortex [33]. These methods provided convincing evidence that changes in activity of part of the brain are accompanied by appropriate changes in its blood flow.

It has been possible to determine local oxygen consumption by the use of $^{15}O_2$ and to correlate local oxygen consumption with regional blood flow in the same area [86]. A good linear correlation was found between these two variables in normal subjects. Although we have used only global methods to determine the cerebral metabolic rate of oxygen consumption ($CMRO_2$) in coma, uncoupling of cerebral metabolism and blood flow may occur; $CMRO_2$ is decreased proportionally to the depth of coma. However, CBF may be low (coupling), normal, or even abnormally high (uncoupling) in traumatic coma.

The mechanisms by which metabolism influences cerebral blood flow are still controversial. There is slight evidence that neuronal reflex mechanisms may be involved [85], but it is more generally accepted that the release of vasodilator metabolites from the active nerve cell is responsible for the coupling between cerebral functional activity and metabolism, on one hand, and cerebral vessel diameter and blood flow, on the other. The identity of the metabolites which function as mediators in metabolic regulation of brain blood flow is uncertain. Promising candidates are adenosine and adenosine phosphorylated derivatives, potassium, hydrogen ion, calcium, and carbon dioxide. A reduction in tissue pO_2 may also contribute to vasodilation during increases in metabolism. This assumption is mainly based on the observation that superfusion of the brain surface with fluorocarbons and a high concentration of oxygen reduced the vasodilation during seizures, but that fluorocarbons equilibrated with nitrogen did not attenuate vasodilation [43].

Knowledge of the state of coupling or uncoupling between cerebral metabolism and blood flow and an understanding of the mechanisms of this coupling is important in the study and treatment of head injury. Vasodilation may lead to increased intracranial pressure (ICP) more than an increase in cerebral edema. Moreover, our most important treatment of high ICP, i.e., hyperventilation, leads to vasoconstriction and a decrease in cerebral blood flow.

If the systemic arterial pressure is lowered or raised quickly, cerebral blood flow falls or increases passively with the change in arterial pressure. Blood flow then returns to the control value within a few seconds when pressure autoregulation is intact. When autoregulation is impaired but still present, the adjustment of blood flow is slower and less complete; and when autoregulation is absent, blood flow passively follows changes in systemic arterial pressure. Thus, autoregulation is a quantitative, measurable variable in the control of the cerebral circulation and not an all-or-nothing phenomenon.

The lower limit of pressure autoregulation to changes in mean systemic arterial pressure is approximately 50 mmHg; the upper limit is about 160 mmHg. This means that as the arterial pressure is decreased, the resistance vessels dilate until they are maximally dilated in response to the decreased perfusion pressure. At a mean pressure of about 50 mmHg, blood flow declines steeply with a further decrease in pressure. When arterial pressure is increased, the vessels constrict until the mean arterial pressure exceeds 160 mmHg, at which point the pressure breaks through the vasoconstriction, causing passive dilation and an increase in cerebral blood flow. Vital dyes usually enter the brain at the moment of breakthrough, manifesting disruption of he blood-brain barrier (BBB) [20]. Presumably, this is a pressure phenomenon within capillaries and small arterioles — the barrier leaks because of a sudden distention of a vessel within the microcirculation. If autoregulation is impaired by hypoxia [3], hypercarbia [32], or minimal blunt trauma to the exposed surface of the brain [88], and the blood pressure is then raised quickly, not only is there extravasation of protein-bound dyes into the brain, but the brain swells acutely and often massively [61].

Apart from vessel diameter changes in response to arterial blood pressure changes, pressure autoregulation is also operative during changes in intracranial pressure. When ICP was increased in experimental animals, blood flow was found to autoregulate in much the same fashion as when systemic arterial pressure was decreased [65]. At lower values of cerebral perfusion pressure (CPP), an increase in ICP was found to be a somewhat more potent stimulator of autoregulatory vasodilation than a decrease in arterial pressure. CPP is generally defined as the difference between mean arterial pressure (MAP) and mean intracranial pressure (CPP = MAP - ICP), but this is not completely true. In fact, the cerebral perfusion pressure is the difference between arterial and cerebral venous pressure, which provides the driving force for flow of blood through the cerebral vascular bed. The difference between intravascular and intracranial pressure at any point within the cerebral circulation gives the transmural pressure which determines the distention of cerebral vessels. Because in humans the cerebral venous pressure is difficult to measure and because it runs practically parallel with ICP, we will assume here, too, that cerebral perfusion pressure equals mean arterial blood pressure minus intracranial pressure.

Either of two mechanisms has been considered to be responsible for pressure autoregulation. The oldest is the myogenic theory, first proposed by Bayliss in 1902 to explain the regulation of the circulation of muscle and other organs and tissues [6]. According to this myogenic hypothesis, the resistance vessels have a high degree of resting vasoconstrictor tone due mainly to smooth muscle contraction in the walls. An increased intraluminal pressure stimulates a further increase in tone by stretching the muscles and causing a reactive shortening of radial fibers and a reduction in vascular diameter. A decrease in intraluminal pressure has the opposite effect. Several objections can be made to this theory. The first is that an increase in intracranial pressure does not lead to stretching of the smooth muscles in the vessel wall so that, in order to contract, the muscle should have some sort of receptor sensitive to the transmural pressure. The second objection is that if venous pressure is raised, which leads to a decrease in CPP but with some increase in arteriolar pressure, the arterioles do not constrict, but dilate [87]. The third objection is that blood viscosity autoregulation, in which no change of pressure occurs at all, seems to be closely related to pressure autoregulation [69,72].

The other mechanism held responsible for pressure autoregulation is metabolic in nature and is based on the premise that the activity of vascular muscle is influenced by vasodilator metabolic products that are produced by surrounding tissue. Based on direct measurement of their concentration during changes in blood pressure, it is unlikely that hydrogen ion or potassium are mediators for pressure autoregulation. During decreases in CPP there is no change in extracellular fluid pH in the immediate vicinity of arterioles, nor is there a change in concentration of potassium [83,102]. Prostaglandins do not seem to be involved [84].

Adenosine is now considered to be the most likely substance to mediate pressure autoregulatory responsiveness. Adenosine concentration in rat brain increases during moderate reduction in arterial pressure [105]. Intra-arterial administration of theophylline, which inhibits the vasodilatory effect of adenosine, virtually abolished the decrease in cerebral vascular resistance observed during hypotension [74]. Theophylline administration during normotension had the opposite effect, causing a decrease in vascular resistance. Adenosine is generated in response to tissue hypoxia [104], so that the final determinant of pressure autoregulation is the amount of oxygen transported to the capillaries. It is also important to note that adenosine is present or can be generated in large amounts by perivascular astrocytes [45,93], so that it seems that functioning neurons are not strictly necessary for pressure autoregulation. In fact, we have found pressure autoregulation to be perfectly intact sometimes, with virtually nonfunctioning cerebral hemispheres (complete absence of cortical evoked potentials).

Blood viscosity autoregulation was shown by us to be present in cats [71]. We reasoned that mannitol, by decreasing blood viscosity, would tend to enhance cerebral blood flow, but that cerebral vessels would constrict to keep CBF relatively constant in a manner analogous to pressure autoregulation. We used the cranial window technique to measure in vivo arteriolar diameters, together with blood viscosity and ICP changes after an intravenous bolus of 1 g/kg body weight of mannitol. Blood viscosity decreased immediately; the greatest decrease (23%) occurred at 10 minutes, and at 75 minutes there was a "rebound" increase of 10%. Vessel diameters decreased concomitantly, the largest decrease being 12% at 10 minutes, which was exactly the same as the 12% decrease in diameter associated with pronounced hyperventilation in the same vessels. At 75 minutes, vessel diameter increased by 12%. ICP changed concomitantly with vessel diameter changes. The correlation between blood viscosity and vessel diameter and ICP was very high. In subsequent papers we were able to confirm the relation between pressure autoregulation and blood viscosity autoregulation [69,72].

With autoregulation intact in normal cats or head-injured patients, changes in blood pressure and changes in blood viscosity were not followed by changes in CBF. With autoregulation defective, either in cats with an acutely occluded middle cerebral artery or in severely head injured patients, lower blood pressure and increased blood viscosity caused lower CBF, while higher blood pressure and decreased blood viscosity were both followed by increased CBF [69]. Moreover, in the head injured patients, it could be shown that the changes in ICP accompanying the blood pressure or blood viscosity alteration with intact autoregulation were concomitant with the assumed changes in CBV. These new findings are important because they show that the effect of mannitol or other so-called osmotic agents may not be mediated only by extraction of extracellular brain water to the intravascular component, but also by changes in blood viscosity and cerebrovascular reactivity. Moreover, they may stimulate the search for new ways of modulating ICP and increasing oxygen availability to the brain [73].

THE EFFECT OF CARBON DIOXIDE AND HYDROGEN ION ON CEREBRAL VESSELS

Carbon dioxide and hydrogen ion have a pronounced relaxing effect on cerebral vascular muscle. Consequently, changes in concentration of CO_2 or changes in pH strongly influence cerebral blood flow, vascular resistance, and, last but not least, cerebral blood volume (CBV). The effect of changes in arterial blood CO_2 tension on cerebral blood flow is pronounced, easily demonstrable, and very consistent.

Low pH relaxes cerebral vascular muscle in vitro and high pH contracts the muscle. Topical application of solution with low pH on the brain surface produces pial arteriolar dilation, and application of solution with high pH produces constriction. This response was obtained when changes in pH were induced by changes in CO_2 at constant bicarbonate ion concentration [41,43] or when changes in bicarbonate ion concentration were made at constant pCO_2 [101]. Application of solutions with markedly varying pCO_2 or bicarbonate ion concentration had no effect on arteriolar diameter unless the pH was allowed to change. Thus, the effect of CO_2 is mediated through changes in extracellular fluid pH. Molecular CO_2 and bicarbonate ion do not have intrinsic vasoactivity. Arteriolar dilation in response to low pH takes place rapidly with a time constant less than 10 seconds.

All of the above vascular responses to changes in pH only take place if the pH alteration is on the side of the CSF and not on the intravascular side. Among the various normal constituents of the blood — such as hydrogen ion, lactic acid, bicarbonate ion, and CO_2 — only changes in arterial concentration of CO_2 lead to rapid cerebral vascular response. This is because only the non-ionized CO_2 molecule can rapidly cross the BBB in either direction. Thus, only changes in arterial CO_2 concentration are rapidly reflected in changes in extracellular CO_2 and, hence, in extracellular pH.

In addition to its direct action on cerebral vascular smooth muscle mediated by changes in extracellular fluid pH, CO_2 may affect cerebral blood flow by other mechanisms. Most prominent of these are its effects on brain metabolism and sympathetic activity. However, reports on the alternative explanations for the effect of CO_2 on the cerebrovascular bed conflict and so will not be discussed further here. Suffice it to say that any effect of CO_2 on the cerebral circulation mediated other than by influence upon extracellular pH is not nearly as important, quantitatively, as the aforementioned direct effect.

There are some indications that prolonged hypocapnia causes a change in responsiveness of cerebral blood flow to acute alterations in $PaCO_2$. However, we have found that when cerebral blood flow was measured at different concentrations of arterial CO_2 after several days of profound hyperventilation, the changes in CBF were the same as those measured in the same patients several days earlier. These later findings seem to indicate that even after several days of hyperventilation, this remains a good means of reducing intracranial pressure. If hyperventilation was no longer effective, this would not necessarily indicate that the cerebral vessels, per se, were not responsive to changes in extracellular pH, but rather that other factors may have played a role here. Although there are indications that diffuse cerebral edema may at times play a role after human head injury [30], it is less likely that diffuse cerebral edema would be caused by a generalized disruption of the blood-brain barrier.

CEREBRAL BLOOD FLOW, CEREBRAL BLOOD VOLUME, AND INTRACRANIAL PRESSURE

According to the Monro-Kellie doctrine, ICP is determined by any one of three intracranial constituents: brain tissues (glia, nerve cells, intracellular and extracellular water), blood (contained in the vessels), and cerebrospinal fluid.

The contribution of the blood to total volume can be estimated at 4 to 4.5 ml/100 g of brain tissue [46,47,95]. Although no figures are available concerning the distribution of the blood over the various parts of the vascular bed, it seems safe to assume that 60% is on the venous side and 40% on the arterial side. Theoretically, the venous system could be compressed if high intracranial pressure prevailed; however, so long as there is outflow of blood, the intravenous pressure must be greater than ICP, so clinically, the venous system is non-compressible. We have found, using the cranial window technique, that the venous diameter does not change in response to blood pressure, blood viscosity, or $PaCO_2$ changes (unpublished data). Thus, all cerebral vascular reactivity is confined to the arterial system, which makes up less than 2% of all intracranial contents, or approximately 25 ml in the adult brain. However, it has been found that with hypocarbia or hypercarbia, arteriolar diameter can decrease 20% or increase 65%, respectively [103]. Because diameters are represented to the second power in the formula defining volume ($V = \pi \times r^2$), these diameter changes lead to a 36% decrease or 172% increase in arterial blood volume, which can be anywhere between 16 and 68 ml. A volume change of only 1 ml can alter ICP by 7 to 8 mmHg in pathological circumstances [64], and it can easily be seen what an enormous impact changes in vessel diameter and CBV may have on ICP.

Although CBF and CBV changes are positively correlated in the case of $PaCO_2$ changes, this is not the case with changes in other parameters. Thus, with blood pressure or blood viscosity changes, CBF may remain relatively constant so long as autoregulation is present and the limits of autoregulation are not exceeded, but CBV is altered. If, for instance, blood pressure drops below the limits of autoregulation, CBF will be decreased with maximal vasodilation still present and consequently increased CBV.

There may even be opposite changes in different parts of the vascular bed. It has been shown that spasm of the angiographically visible arteries after subarachnoid hemorrhage with decreased blood flow can lead to an increase in CBF, presumably due to maximal dilation of the vascular bed behind the spastic artery [31].

We conclude that although CBV and ICP are positively correlated, CBV and CBF are only positively correlated under certain circumstances and therefore the relation between CBF and ICP is not easily defined.

The [133]Xenon Method for Measuring Regional CBF

The technique of measuring CBF with freely diffusible radioisotopes was developed by Lassen and Ingvar and began to receive wide clinical application in the late 1960s [55]. A bolus of the radioactive isotope ^{133}Xe dissolved in saline was injected through an indwelling catheter into the internal carotid artery. Most head-injured patients have had cerebral angiography prior to the CBF measurements, and ordinarily the CBF study had been carried out in the hemisphere with the most evidence of lateralized brain damage. As the bolus of injected ^{133}Xe enters the intracranial circulation, the isotope diffuses rapidly through the brain tissue. Since the xenon is largely cleared from the body during one circulation through the lungs, blood reaching the brain after bolus injection is nearly completely free of the isotope. However, the clearance of ^{133}Xe from the cerebral tissue can be recorded with multiple scintillation detectors mounted in a lead collimator block which is placed adjacent to the patient's head. The number of detectors can range from a few to more than 200.

When the isotope enters the cerebral circulation, there is an almost instantaneous rise in the gamma emission recorded by all detectors, and this constitutes the height of the CBF clearance curve. The number of counts diminishes over time and the area underneath the clearance curve is measured for 10 or 15 minutes. CBF is then calculated as the ratio of the height over the area. However, a good estimate of CBF can also be obtained from the "initial slope" of the first two minutes of the clearance curve. Normally, the clearance curve contains two compartments: a fast-flow compartment, believed to represent gray matter, and a slower compartment with about one quarter of the flow of the first compartment, believed to represent white matter. Recent data have made it very questionable, however, if fast- and slow-flow compartments indeed represent gray and white matter, respectively [56]. In patients with brain injuries, the first compartment may contain very fast flows, which are defined as hyperemia or, on the contrary, CBF may be markedly reduced to the point that the curve is nonexponential; i.e., white matter and gray matter flows from that region are now indistinguishable. Toward the completion of a CBF study, the gamma emission from the brain approaches the background of radioactivity in the study room, but another CBF study can be carried out, generally about half an hour after the first run.

The major disadvantages of the intracarotid ^{133}Xe methodology are the need to puncture the carotid artery in order to introduce the isotope and the fact that CBF is recorded only from one hemisphere. Most investigators have concluded that intracarotid CBF studies are justified only in patients who are undergoing carotid angiography for diagnostic purposes. Furthermore, only a few studies can be done at one session for fear that the indwelling carotid catheter in place for a long period of time may lead to serious complications. With the advent of CT scanning of the brain, it became apparent that the indications for cerebral angiography during acute stages of head injury would be limited and, indeed, the CT scanner has largely eliminated the need for angiography in acute head injuries. This meant that the opportunities for measuring CBF in head-injured patients would be extremely limited. Fortunately, the development of the noninvasive methodology for administering the ^{133}Xe has permitted continuation of studies of the cerebral circulation, not only in head-injured patients but in a wide variety of other neurological conditions where the invasive technique was no longer justified.

The noninvasive technique most widely used today is the inhalation methodology developed by Obrist et al [77], modified so as to introduce the ^{133}Xe by intravenous injection as recommended by Austin et al [5]. In our studies of head-injured patients, a 30 mCi bolus of ^{133}Xe is injected intravenously or the patient breathes a gas mixture containing 10 mCi/l of ^{133}Xe for one minute. Radioactivity is monitored for 15 minutes by 16 scintillation detectors, 8 over each hemisphere. The clearance curves are subjected to a two-compartment computer analysis that employs a correction for recirculation based on isotope concentration in the expired air. This provides estimates of blood flow from the faster-clearing or first compartment (F1) and from the slower-clearing or second compartment (F2). Because of the instability of compartmental analysis in patients with severe intracranial pathology [78], a second blood flow index (CBF 15 or CBF infinity) is also calculated. This index represents the mean flow of all tissues seen by the detector, including a small extracerebral component and, unlike F1, it is relatively insensitive to shifts in compartment size [78]. CBF_{15} and CBF_{inf} are different in that in CBF_{15}, the tail of the washout curve is cut off at 15 minutes, thus neglecting the slowest clearing compartments. The disadvantage of the CBF_{inf} method is that at normal flows possibly too much of the skin flow is included, leading to an underestimation of CBF. However, at very low flow, the CBF_{inf} is probably more accurate than CBF_{15}. At very high flows, the contribution of the very slow clearing compartments becomes negligible. However, these differences are minor and in this report we have considered these flow indices to be similar and they are both referred to as CBF_{15}. In most cases in this report, the value of CBF_{15} found at the prevailing $PaCO_2$ was recalculated to a normative $PaCO_2$ of 34 mmHg, assuming a 3% change in CBF per 1 mmHg change in $PaCO_2$ [76]. The 3% change per torr CO_2 was non-compounded (for instance to convert a CBF_{15} value of 50 ml/100 gm/min at $PaCO_2 = 29$ mmHg, we simply added $(34 - 29) \times 3\% \times 50 = 7.5$ ml/100 gm/min to obtain 58 ml/100 gm/min at $PaCO_2 - 34$ mmHg) $PaCO_2 = 34$ mmHg was chosen because most measurements were performed at this approximate value. Reducing CBF_{15} values to a normative value at $PaCO_2 = 34$ mmHg makes them more readily comparable to each other. This CBF value is designated CBF(34) and is clearly indicated as such where applicable. Normal CBF(34) in young adults is 44.1 ± 5.6(SD) ml/100 gm/min [76]. The data are analyzed by computer in the head injury clinical unit or intensive care unit, with hard copy printouts of results available within 5 minutes of completion of the CBF study.

In some patients, the administration of the large doses of xenon gas (between 30% and 50% of inhaled gases) lead to increased ICP, presumably the result of a direct vasodilatatory effect of the gas in this concentration. This may not only be dangerous for the patient, it may also lead to underestimation of low flows which are increased with vasodilatation.

Measurements of AVDO$_2$ and CMRO$_2$

In approximately two thirds of our patients in the present report, a catheter was placed in the jugular bulb through retrograde cannulation of the right internal jugular vein for measuring arteriovenous difference of oxygen (AVDO$_2$). AVDO$_2$ was calculated from arterial and jugular venous oxygen content. Oxygen content was evaluated by a direct oximetry. During the CBF measurements, two arterial and jugular samples were taken for AVDO$_2$ measurement and the average of these two measurements was used for calculation of cerebral metabolic rate of oxygen (CMRO$_2$) – CMRO$_2$ = CBF $\times$ AVDO$_2$/100. Normal AVDO$_2$ is 6.4 $\pm$ 1.2 vol% and normal CMRO$_2$ is 3.2 ml/100 g/min [39]. In some cases values of AVDO$_2$ were, just as CBF, normalized to a value at PaCO$_2$ of 34 torr. A change of 3% per torr change in PaCO$_2$ was assumed just as with CBF, but of course in the opposite direction. Normal AVDO$_2$ at PaCO$_2$ 34 mmHg would be 6.3 + (6 $\times$ 3% $\times$ 6.3) = 7.4 vol%.

Rationale for CBF Studies after severe head injury

Langfitt and Obrist have defined several purposes for clinical cerebral blood flow studies [49]. The first is to determine if CBF is sufficient to meet the metabolic demands of the brain. Although coma itself can reduce hemispheric metabolism by some 40%, there is a basic metabolism which must be maintained to provide integrity of the cells [4]. Thus, there is a threshold of flow under which even basic metabolism cannot be maintained and the cells disintegrate. This threshold has not been exactly determined and it is also duration-dependent and possibly species-dependent. However, it seems that focal ischemic infarction occurs almost immediately with flows of 7 ml/100 g/minute, with flows of 10 to 12 ml after 2 to 3 hours, and even with flows of 17 to 18 ml if permanent [36].

A second purpose of measuring CBF after severe head injury has been to evaluate its usefulness in predicting the clinical outcome. Up until now, CBF has had only very limited use for this purpose. Because multimodality evoked potentials (MEPs) may better suit this goal [29], in certain circumstances the two methods may usefully be combined, especially if CMRO$_2$ is used instead of plain CBF [89].

A third purpose of the CBF studies has been to assess the responsiveness of the cerebral circulation by testing autoregulation and by evaluating cerebrovascular reactivity to changes in PaCO$_2$. One hypothesis that has served as a stimulus for these studies has been that the responses of CBF to changes in blood pressure or PaCO$_2$ might be predictive of outcome, even though the level of CBF at the time of the initial study and its subsequent course were not of prognostic value. Moreover, cerebrovascular reactivity may be closely linked to ICP changes, the latter being thought of as an important parameter in head injury.

Finally, the most important reason for measuring cerebral blood flow and metabolism has been to evaluate various therapeutic regimens. For example, if it could be found that CBF is reduced to a level well below metabolism or the infraction threshold and that, in turn, CBF can be increased by a particular therapeutic agent, this observation would dictate that this therapy should be continued and repeat measurements of CBF be performed in order to determine if the agent continues to be effective or still necessary over time. It might be argued that if therapy is beneficial, the benefit will be manifested by improvements in the patient's neurological status and therefore measurements of CBF and metabolism are of little use; but it is likely that the beneficial therapy would have to be continued for a long period before clear improvement in the neurologic status becomes evident [49].

Moreover, because of the many variables in head injury, it takes an extraordinarily large number of patients before any specific therapy can be proven to be beneficial. However, by identifying the subgroups who need a given therapy and by demonstrating its direct effect other than outcome, it becomes much easier to test new modes of therapy.

Consequently, the following questions need to be addressed:

1. Does very low CBF play a role in determining clinical status and outcome?
2. Does very high CBF play a role in ICP elevation?
3. How can CBF be manipulated (autoregulation, CO_2 reactivity, mannitol) as well as effects on other parameters such as clinical status, ICP, pressure volume index (PVI), multimodality evoked potentials, and, finally, outcome?

Sufficiency of CBF After Head Injury

The first of the purposes of measuring CBF in severe head injuries as defined by Langfitt and Obrist was to determine if CBF is sufficient to meet the metabolic demands of the brain [49]. For several reasons, this question is very difficult to answer. First of all, it is not known what the cerebral demands after head injury really are. Also, if areas of the brain are disrupted by the impact itself, they won't recover function whether metabolic demands are met by CBF or not. Thus, even very low flows may not alter outcome and higher flows would be of no use to the damaged brain anyway. One way to try to find an answer to this question would be by separating primary inflicted and secondary ischemic damage. In humans, only the Glasgow group claims to have found clear ischemic damage in head-injured patients [2,28,35]. Interestingly, most ischemic changes were found in the frontal-parietal "watershed" area where Overgaard and co-workers found the largest number of regions with very low flows (less than 17 m/100 g/min) [81]. These findings occurred only in patients who did poorly. In this last study, 35 probes over one hemisphere were used after intracarotid delivery of the [133]xenon, resulting in a very high resolution; and even with a number of areas with flows below 17 or 20 ml/100 g/min, global hemispheric flow (CBF_{10}, height-over-area method) was sometimes well over 30 ml/100 g/min [81]. Thus, with the much smaller number (eight) of probes per hemisphere that we

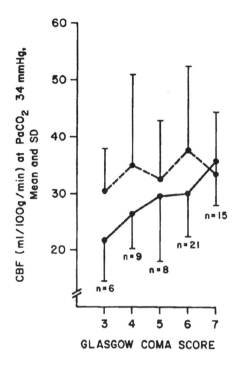

Figure 4.1. Relationship between Glasgow Coma Score and Cerebral Blood Flow (CBF$_{15}$ at PaCO$_2$ 34 mmHg) in patients older than 18 years. Solid line: measurements taken within 12 hours after injury. Broken line: measurements in the same patients 24 to 48 hours after injury.

use, it is not likely that we will be able to find the same result and we know of no other reports which allow us to make this correlation between pathologic findings and CBF measurements.

If one assumes that clinical condition is related to the level of CBF, one would expect lower CBF with lower Glasgow Coma Score (GCS). However, in almost none of the many papers on CBF after head injury could such a relationship be established. Only Yoshino and co-workers found the lowest CBF values in the patients with the worst clinical condition, and on the side of the brain with the most severe damage on CT scanning [107]. It is noteworthy that these authors were able to perform their flow measurements within three hours of the trauma, as opposed to the usual "within the 1st to 10th day" of most other papers. We have correlated the average CBF$_{15}$ of both hemispheres at PaCO$_2$ 34 mmHg with the GCS in 59 patients in whom measurements could be performed within 12 hours post-injury. These patients are all 19 years of age or older and form exactly half of 118 adult patients on whom CBF measurements were done at the Medical College of Virginia in Richmond. Results are shown in Figure 4.1. Obviously, there is a trend for higher flows with better coma scores, which is also statistically significant (ANOVA – test $p < 0.01$). It should be noted, however, the SDs are fairly large, so that in individual cases it is not possible to relate CBF and clinical condition. In the other 59 adult patients, in whom the first

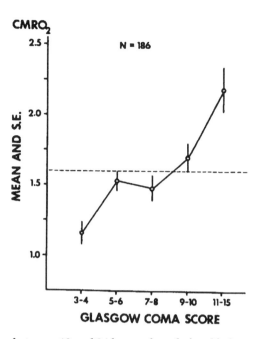

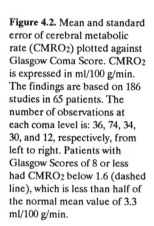

Figure 4.2. Mean and standard error of cerebral metabolic rate (CMRO2) plotted against Glasgow Coma Score. CMRO2 is expressed in ml/100 g/min. The findings are based on 186 studies in 65 patients. The number of observations at each coma level is: 36, 74, 34, 30, and 12, respectively, from left to right. Patients with Glasgow Scores of 8 or less had CMRO2 below 1.6 (dashed line), which is less than half of the normal mean value of 3.3 ml/100 g/min.

measurement was usually taken between 12 and 24 hours, the relationship between CBF and GCS is already lost, while in the whole group with measurements after 24 hours, there is no relation whatsoever between CBF and GCS or motor score. The conclusion from these and Yoshino's data must be that early after injury (< 12 hours) CBF and GCS are related. This could not be established in other reports because CBF measurements were done after that relationship had already disappeared, even though the other investigations were done in "the acute state" after head injury. Of course, a positive relation between CBF and clinical condition does not prove any causal relationship, but it is, at least, compatible with such a contention.

In Figure 4.2, the relationship between the CMRO2 and Glasgow Coma Score is shown, as measured in 186 occasions in 65 patients [76]. It shows a clear relation between CMRO2 and clinical condition but, again, we cannot conclude from such a relationship that the low CMRO2 is the cause of the low coma score. Another way to look at this is to see if the brain extracted more than a normal amount of O2 per unit of blood when blood flow was low. In Figure 4.3, the arteriovenous difference of oxygen is shown for patients with reduced flow or with hyperemia (as defined by Obrist et al [76]). The normal range of AVDO2 is 6 to 6.9 and it can be seen that only one patient had a much larger difference, indicating a (relative) ischemia and 7 patients had a slightly increased AVDO2. Even with reduced flow, many patients (fifteen) had a decreased AVDO2, indicating that blood flow was probably in excess of metabolic demands. This makes it unlikely that low CBF per se is, at the point measured, the cause of the clinical condition. However, Table 4.1 shows the results

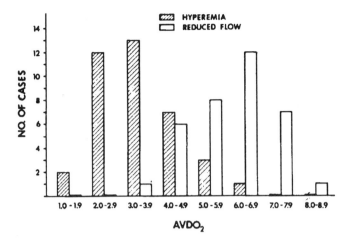

Figure 4.3. Cerebral arteriovenous oxygen differences (AVDO2) expressed in vol% for two groups of head-injured patients classified according to CBF. Patients with reduced flow had normal AVDO2 while those with hyperemia had significantly lower values.

Table 4.1. Wide Arteriovenous Oxygen Differences (9-12 vol%) Induced by Hyperventilation

	Mean ± SD*	
	10 Hyperventilated Patients	Normal Value (PaCO2 40)
CMRO2	1.9 ± 0.5	3.3 ±0.4
CBF15	18.6 ±4.4	53.3 ± 6.8
AVDO2	10.5 ± 0.7	6.3 ± 1.2
VpO2	22.3 ± 1.8	37.5 ± 5.6

Occurrence: 10 out of 55 patients. Time Post-Injury: 10-85 hours. Glasgow Coma Score: 4-9 (Mean = 6.4). PaCO2 (Mean ± SD) = 23.2 ± 2.8 mmHg
*CMRO2 and CBF15 are expressed in ml/100 g/min; AVDO2 is vol%; VpO2 is in mmHg.

of measurements of CBF, CMRO2, and AVDO2 during the test of hyperventilation. Under those circumstances, AVDO2 rose above 9 volume percent in 10 out of 55 patients, showing that those patients were on the brink of ischemia. The conclusion must be that vigorous hyperventilation may, in a certain but yet unknown percentage of patients, lead to the development of ischemia. In practice, this means that one must be somewhat cautious with the use of very vigorous hyperventilation. In non-research centers, CBF measurements in these patients may not easily be obtained, but AVDO2 can be used as a guideline instead.

Yet another way to investigate the relationship between clinical conditions and ischemia is by increasing CBF in those patients in whom it seems to be insufficient (CBF15 less than 18 ml/100 g/min, or AVDO2 greater than 9 vol%, or both). Brown and co-workers have treated rhesus monkeys with mannitol after an experimental missile injury [8,15,16]. In the untreated group, CBF fell to a minimum of 16 ml/100 g/min (initial slope method after [133]xenon injection in one internal carotid artery). This drop was prevented to a large extent by mannitol, with a concomitant improvement in $CMRO_2$ above 2 ml/100 g/min, from 1.5 ml/100 g/min in the untreated animals. The $CMRO_2$ value of 1.5 ml/100 g/min in the untreated animals closely approaches the supposedly critical value of 1.4, under which membrane failure appears, leading to structural cell damage [4]. This is similar to the $CMRO_2$ value of 1.5 ml/100 g/min found by Roquefeuil et al as an important threshold for survival after head injury in man [89]. Also, the six-hour survival in the treated group was much higher than in the untreated group. It is true that other parameters such as ICP, blood pressure, and cerebral perfusion pressure also improved, but the improvement in CBF was out of proportion to the changes in these parameters. Although another direct effect from mannitol cannot be ruled out, we have concluded from the work of Brown and co-workers that it is the increased CBF (and secondary $CMRO_2$) which improves outcome in these animals. It should be noted that ischemia in these animals was treated within 15 to 60 minutes after injury.

Similar data after human head injuries are virtually nonexistent. In 150 patients studied within the first 24 hours by one of us, 12 (8%) were found to have CBF values below 18 ml/100 g/min, regardless of $PaCO_2$. A couple of patients with very high ICP and low CPP causing "ischemia" are not considered here. In 7 of those 12 patients, we also have $AVDO_2$ values: 5 were well below 8 vol%, indicating that the brain was not extracting a larger than normal amount of oxygen out of the little blood flowing through it. Thus in these cases, the low CBF was merely a reflection of very low metabolism. In one patient, $AVDO_2$ was 8.3 vol%, compatible with borderline ischemia, but when his blood pressure was raised to obtain an increase of CBF from 16 to 34 ml/100 g/min, $AVDO_2$ decreased to 4.4 vol%, keeping $CMRO_2$ almost unchanged. His somatosensory evoked potentials, which are considered a sensitive indication of ischemia [15,62,91], and visual evoked potentials also did not change with raising of his CBF. Only one of the 7 "ischemic" patients with $AVDO_2$ measurements showed a very high value of 11.6 vol%. In this case, we raised his blood pressure and hyperventilated less to raise his $PaCO_2$ from 28 to 34 mmHg; these two maneuvers raised his CBF from 15 to 32 ml/100 g/min, and even though his $AVDO_2$ dropped from 11.6 to 7.7 vol%, his $CMRO_2$ increased from 1.74 to 2.45 ml/100 g/min. At the same time, an immediate improvement in his somatosensory evoked potentials was seen, consisting of decreased central conduction time and increased late wave amplitude and complexity. In this case we must assume that the patient was really ischemic at the time of his first $AVDO_2$ and CBF measurement 8 hours post-injury. At later measurements, 16, 42, and 89 hours post-injury, no low CBF or high $AVDO_2$ values were found. In 5 patients with CBF below 18 ml/100 g/min, we do not have $AVDO_2$ measurements. Four of those have been described earlier, and we concluded that because of improvements in clinical condition and evoked potential parameters, 3 of the 4 were ischemic in the sense of CBF not being able to support metabolism [67,68]. In the other patient, and in the one not described earlier, we do not believe that CBF was below the demands of cerebral metabolism at the time of the measurements. In summary, in the first 24 hours post-injury, we found 12 out of 150 patients (8%) with normal CPP who had CBF below the threshold of 18 ml/100 g/min for ischemia; but in only 4 (3%) do we have clear indications that cerebral metabolism and function — clinically and electrically — were depressed because of ischemia. After 24 hours, there were only 2 such patients.

A conclusion must be drawn from this data that ischemia does play a distinct, but very small, role in determining clinical status and outcome after severe head injuries, so far as we have been able to determine. Whether ischemia occurs much more often very shortly after injury is a question which can be reasonably answered in laboratory investigations only. In this respect it is also interesting to note that Brown and co-workers could improve outcome in their most severely injured monkeys only if treatment of ischemia was begun within 15 minutes post-injury [8,15,16].

At this time we can only speculate about the reason for ischemia as found by us. One possible explanation is that of vasospasm in the large conducting, angiographically visible, vessels, as has been shown to occur in about 19% of a group of 350 patients with severe, but also with moderately severe, head injuries in which angiography of one or both carotids was performed between 0 and 39 days post-injury [60,97].

In one of our patients with low CBF and large AVDO2, angiography did show vasospasm. The assumption of vasospasm could also explain why ICP is not raised to a large extent with induced hypertension. With normotension there is only a minimal hydrostatic pressure in the microcirculation, which vessels may even be maximally dilated to compensate for low local perfusion pressure as has been postulated to occur in vasospasm after subarachnoid hemorrhage from aneurysmal rupture [31]. Overcoming resistance in the larger but spastic arteries only leads to restoration of perfusion pressure in the microcirculation toward normal. Thus, the fear that hypertension after trauma might induce high ICP [63] or enhance cerebral edema [61] is not warranted in all cases. Thus it may not be advantageous to arbitrarily "stabilize" that MAP at a lower level without knowledge of CBF or AVDO2.

We have found it feasible to treat ischemia after severe head injury with induced hypertension in much the same way as after subarachnoid hemorrhage [66,69]. If vasospasm is indeed the cause for ischemia as we found, it still may be completely different from "vasospasm" after subarachnoid hemorrhage. Therefore it may be worthwhile to treat it with drugs that can dilate spastic cerebral vessels, such as Ca^{2+} channel blockers. However, the role played by ischemia after severe head injury needs further elucidation and the best way to pursue this is by early and frequent CBF and AVDO2 measurements, combined with studies of evoked potentials.

Hyperemia and Elevated ICP

As mentioned above, the relationship between CBF and CBV and, thus, ICP is not a linear one and, in fact, may be reversed in a number of cases. Increased CBV

Table 4.2. CBF Findings in Two Groups of Head Injured Patients Classified According to ICP*

	No. of Cases	
Acute CBF Findings	ICP > 20 mmHG	ICP < 20 mmHg
Hyperemia (n = 14)	27 (77%)	14 (100%)
Reduced flow (n = 34)	8 (23%)	26 (65%)
Total (n = 75)	35 (100%)	40 (100%)

*The two ICP groups differed significantly with respect to CBF (p < 0.001, chi-square test).

can safely be assumed to be present only in cases with very high CBF, irrespective of $PaCO_2$; in all other cases it may or may not be present. Nevertheless, a great deal of attention has been drawn to the occurrence of elevated ICP concomitant with hyperemia, especially in children [9,11]. Bruce et al argue that in children, hyperemia is the chief cause of elevated ICP. The very good results obtained by this group in the treatment of head-injured children were ascribed specifically to the generous use of hyperventilation to decrease CBF and CBV, resulting in excellent control of ICP. Because mannitol, which is widely used to decrease elevated ICP, had been shown to increase CBF in a number of head-injured patients [10], Bruce's group even goes so far as to dismiss its use in children because it is feared it might lead to increased CBF with secondarily higher ICP [9]. Although we do not believe that their fear is justified, it shows that there is a relationship between ICP and CBF that is not fully understood as yet.

Obrist has noted that hyperemia can not be defined by CBF criteria alone, but that $AVDO_2$ and $CMRO_2$ in relation to the depth of coma must be taken into account as well [76]. $CMRO_2$ is roughly proportional to the depth of coma, and for all patients with GCS 3 to 7 after acute head injury averages approximately half of normal. Since under normal conditions, blood flow is functionally coupled with metabolism, the occurrence of CBF above half of normal CBF suggests an uncoupling of $CMRO_2$ and CBF. Therefore, at a $PaCO_2$ of 34 mmHg, below normal minus 2 SD (under 33 ml/100 g/min) is considered a threshold for reduced flow. CBF values between 33 and 55 ml/100 g/min represent relative hyperemia and above 55 ml/100 g/min represents absolute hyperemia [76].

Obrist et al related the occurrence of increased ICP to the level of CBF in a series of 75 adult patients (age 15 to 85 years, with a median of 28 years) [76]. During the acute illness, 35 patients (47%) developed intracranial hypertension, defined as an ICP greater than 20 mmHg recorded on at least two occasions, but it usually involved sustained or repeated elevations ranging from 20 to 40 mmHg. The remaining 40 cases (53%) did not have intracranial hypertension; that is, their ICP never exceeded 20 mmHg. In classifying the patients, care was taken to exclude spuriously high ICP recordings attributable to suctioning, coughing, gross head movement, or improper transducer calibration.

Table 4.2 presents the CBF findings in these two ICP groups. Whereas 77% of the patients with ICPs greater than 20 mmHg revealed hyperemia, only 23% had a

Table 4.3. ICP and PVI at the Time of CBF Measurements* (Pediatric Patients Only)

	Reduced Flow		Relative Hyperemia		Absolute Hyperemia
	(n = 16)	(n = 8)	(n = 16)	(n = 8)	(n = 20)
CBF(34)	< 32.9	32.9 - 38.3	38.4 - 49.7	49.8 - 55.3	> 55.3
Average ICP	15.3 ± 7.5	12.8 ± 7.1	16.2 ± 4.0	16.9 ± 8.9	15.5 ± 8.2
%ICP > 20 mmHg	29	20	13	25	25
PVI > 18 ml(n)	0	0	2	1	2
PVI < 18 ml(n)	1	0	2	2	6

*CBF (34) is CBF_{15} reduced to $PaCO_2$ of 34 mmHg, assuming a 3% change in CBF per torr change in $PaCO_2$, expressed in ml/100 g/min. ICP in mmHg. Average ICP is mean ± SD. (n) = number.

consistently reduced flow. The reverse trend was found in patients with ICPs below 20 mmHg; 35% showed hyperemia while 65% had a reduced flow. The difference was highly significant statistically.

Although hyperemia was clearly associated with increased ICP, it also occurred in one-third of the patients with normal pressures. It should be noted, however, that many patients in the latter group were being vigorously treated for prevention of intracranial hypertension. In the absence of such therapy, the correlation between hyperemia and increased ICP might have been even higher.

We have performed the same analysis in a series of 32 head-injured pediatric patients (age 3 to 18 years, median 15 years), in which hyperemia is even more common. Table 4.3 shows the average ICP in different CBF groups. ICPs in each of those groups were not significantly different from each other, nor was there a significant trend to have higher ICP with higher blood flow. The percentages of ICP greater than 20 mmHg are also not different in the various groups. Especially in the groups with reduced flows and with absolute hyperemia, they were similar, with 29% in both groups. It should be noted that in the group with reduced flows, two ICP values of respectively 60 and 76 mmHg have been omitted in these calculations. It was thought that in those two occasions, low CBF (16 ml/100 g/min in both cases) was caused by low cerebral perfusion pressure (around 25 mmHg) with uncontrolled ICP as a terminal event; both patients died within hours of these measurements.

We also classified the pediatric patients in two ICP groups: one in which ICP never exceeded 20 mmHg (9 patients, 28%) and another in which ICP exceeded 20 mmHg at some point during the acute phase (23 patients, 72%). Of course, ICP elevations during coughing, suctioning, spuriously high $PaCO_2$, etc., were not considered true elevations here. These two ICP groups were correlated with the occurrence of reduced flow or with hyperemia, using the criteria of Obrist where all flows higher than normal minus two SD is considered hyperemia during a comatose state. These findings are presented in Table 4.4. Due to the very small number of patients with reduced flow, there is no value in statistical testing.

Table 4.4. CBF Findings in Two Groups of Head-Injured Children Classified according to ICP and PVI*

Acute CBF Findings	Total Cases	ICP > 20 mmHg (no.)	ICP < 20 mmHg (no.)	PVI < 18 ml (no.)	PVI > 18 ml (no.)
Hyperemia	28	19	9	10	7
Reduced Flow	4	4	0	1	0
Totals	32	23	9	11	7

*Hyperemia: CBF(34) $\geq$ 33 ml/100 g/min. Reduced flow: CBF(34) < 33 ml/100 g/min.

Although ICP elevations above 20 mmHg, necessitating drainage of CSF or administration of mannitol, were common in this series of pediatric patients, the number of ICP elevations may have been limited as most of the patients were rather vigorously hyperventilated: the average $PaCO_2$ of the measurements at 24 to 48 hours was 27.2 ± 4.6 mmHg; after 48 hours, 25.5 ± 5.4 mmHg. We, therefore, have also looked at pressure-volume-index (PVI) measurements in these children [59]. PVI is an index of brain compliance: the lower the PVI value, the less compliant the brain is. Although normal PVI in children is 25 ml, we have chosen a value of 18 ml as acceptable or "normal" (Marmarou, personal communication, 1987). PVI measurements were performed in 18 of the last 24 children in this series. On 16 occasions, PVI measurement was performed within minutes from the CBF measurement. The relation between the two measurements is shown in Table 4.4. Although low PVI occurred somewhat more often in the group with absolute hyperemia, this was not significant due to the small numbers. PVI remained above an acceptable threshold of 18 ml throughout the first 5 days in 7 of 18 (39%, "normal" PVI group), while it was below normal once (single measurement) or at least twice during this period in the other 11 children (61%, low PVI group). These two PVI groups were divided over the two CBF groups just as was done with ICP, but in only one out of the four patients with consistent reduced flows, PVI measurements were performed, precluding any statistical testing. It is noteworthy that there were 7 patients who were hyperemic at some time in their acute course, in whom PVI remained normal all the time. On the other hand, the three children with the lowest PVI values (around 6 ml) also had consistently the highest flows. Interestingly, all 3 of these children had a favorable outcome.

Several explanations may be forwarded for the discrepancy between the earlier findings in adults and the present findings in children. In the first place, 28 of 32 children in this report were "hyperemic" at some point, making any comparison between those four patients with reduced flow and the group with hyperemia meaningless. In the second place, most of our patients were quite vigorously hyperventilated at the time of the CBF measurement. In all 32 pediatric patients with 73 measurements, the average actual CBF_{15} was only 43.8 ± 21.9 ml/100 g/min. It is true, considering the $AVDO_2$ values (around 4 vol%), that this represents hyperemia in relation to $CMRO_2$; but in an absolute sense, 44 ml/110 g/min is below normal, especially for a group with a mean age of only 13 years (normal CBF_{15} at $PaCO_2$ of 40 mmHg at this age can be estimated at 70 ml/100 g/min). Another problem is that the relation between CBF and CBV (and thus, ICP) is not a linear one; in fact, it is extremely complicated. CBF is determined by MABP and ICP, blood viscosity, and vessel diameter, while CBV is determined by vessel diameter – the latter being the common denominator for both CBF and CBV. Thus while increased vessel diameter will always lead to increased CBV and possibly increased ICP (if compensatory mechanisms have been exhausted), it can be accompanied by high, normal, or even low CBF. So the relationship between CBF and ICP remains uncertain, even though Obrist et al had found that elevated ICP occurred more often with hyperemia. However, the individual variation was large, precluding drawing conclusions in individual cases. Moreover, in the group of pediatric patients presented here in which hyperemia was much more prevalent, these earlier findings could not be confirmed. This may be due in part to a too generous definition of hyperemia. On the other hand, Obrist's prophecy [76] that a measure other than ICP might better correlate with CBF has partly come true: the three children with CBF values even higher than CBF at normal $PaCO_2$ in awake children had the lowest values of PVI, even though they had normal or only moderately elevated ICP.

CEREBROVASCULAR AUTOREGULATION (REACTIVITY) AFTER SEVERE HEAD INJURY

As mentioned above, the cerebral vasculature is regulated by metabolism (metabolic autoregulation), CPP (pressure autoregulation), blood viscosity (blood viscosity autoregulation), and $PaCO_2$ (CO_2 reactivity).

We have shown already that metabolic autoregulation is impaired in most cases with severe head injury. In the few cases with (reversible) ischemia and high $AVDO_2$, the mechanism of metabolic autoregulation may or may not be intact, but blood supply is simply not able to meet metabolic demands. In the case with "ischemia" and normal or low $AVDO_2$ and very low $CMRO_2$ and in the cases with "reduced flow," metabolic autoregulation is assumed to be intact. However in all other cases, cerebral blood flow exceeds demands, and thus there is uncoupling between flow and metabolism. This is most evident in our series of 32 children who show the highest blood flow values: $AVDO_2$ was below 4 vol% in 58% of the measurements! We do not think there is a good explanation for this loss of metabolic autoregulation or uncoupling. It has been suggested that posttraumatic hyperemia, the "luxury perfusion" described by Lassen [54], and the "vasomotor paralysis" described by Langfitt and co-workers [50,51,52] are all related. Lassen considered the "luxury perfusion" after stroke to be due to lactic acidosis. Although high levels of lactic acid have been found in cerebrospinal fluid after head injury in several series of patients [18,21], we and others have been able to find a relations between lactic acid and level of CBF [17,21]. Moreover, in many cases, elevated CSF lactic acid levels return to normal within 48 hours [18], so at the time that hyperemia is maximal, there is probably no longer any lactic acidosis. The cause of "vasomotor paralysis" after experimental brain injury is uncertain. In a cat model with focal brain injury (small cold lesion), we have also found generalized (remote from the injury site) vasodilation and loss of CO_2 reactivity [108]. These changes were at least partly related to oxygen radicals, as they could be prevented by local administration of radical scavengers. However, this vasodilation is fairly short-lived and also CO_2 reactivity returns within a couple of hours. In clinical series, CO_2 reactivity is intact in most cases at the time of the CBF measurements [22,76,79] and we have found that pressure autoregulation is also intact in two-thirds of the patients in the present series. Thus, although there is metabolic uncoupling, the blood vessels in most cases still respond to the normal stimuli of CO_2 or blood pressure changes, which is not in accordance with the concept of vasomotor paralysis.

The data on cerebral perfusion pressure autoregulation remains confusing. In Kasoff's study of children, more regional peaks were found after raising blood pressure, which was taken as an absence of autoregulation [37]. The same was found by Enevoldsen et al in cortical lesions shortly after the injury in patients with so-called brain stem lesions [22]. However, autoregulation was found intact during the first few days and only later deteriorated temporarily. It is not possible to say anything about prognosis from either of these studies. In an earlier study by one of us, there was so much variability in the status of autoregulation among patients and from region to region within the same patient, that no conclusion could be drawn [81]. Two other studies reached two completely opposite conclusions [23,79]. Considering all this, it is not possible to draw any firm conclusion on pressure autoregulation and outcome. However, all these studies precede the use of the Glasgow Coma Score for clinical evaluation and the use of the CT scanner for anatomical correlation. We have now tested autoregulation in 100 severely head-injured patients either by increasing their blood pressure with phenylephrine (which by itself hardly constricts cerebral blood vessels as these have very few alpha adrenergic receptors) or by decreasing blood pressure with trimetaphan-camsylate (Arfonad®), a ganglionic blocker which by itself also does not cause cerebral vasodilation. Part of these results have been presented earlier [69,70] and we will present here only results of autoregulation tests in children. Not only are the results in children basically similar to those in adults, but because of the prevalence of hyperemia in children, they are also somewhat more difficult to understand. For determination of the site of injury, we used multimodality evoked potentials (MEPS) and we divided the children in groups of those with cortical lesions, with diencephalic lesions, with brain stem lesions, or with a combination thereof.

A total of 34 pressure autoregulation tests were performed in 24 children. Autoregulation was found to be intact 21 times (62%) and defective 13 times (38%). Autoregulation was tested by increasing MABP by an average of 29% with phenylephrine on 22 occasions and found to be intact 13 times (59%). Arfonad decreased

Table 4.5. Relation between Autoregulation (Intact or Defective) and Site of Injury as Determined with Multimodality Evoked Potentials* in 24 Pediatric Patients

Autoregulation	Normal	H	B-S	H + D	H + B-S	H + D + B-S	Total
Intact (n)	3	9	3	2	2	2	21
Defective (n)		8			3	2	13

H = Hemispheres; B-S = Brain Stem; D = Diencephalon. (n) = number

Table 4.6. Relation between Autoregulation (Intact or Defective) and the Level of CBF in 24 Pediatric Patients*

Autoregulation	Reduced Flow		Relative Hyperemia		Absolute Hyperemia
CBF (34)	< 32.9	32.9 - 38.3	38.4 - 49.7	49.8 - 55.3	> 55.3
Intact (n)	2	3	7	5	3
Defective (n)	6		3	1	4

*CBF(34) is CBF_{15} reduced to $PaCO_2$ of 34 mmHg, assuming a 3% change in CBF per torr change in $PaCO_2$. (n) = number.

MABP by an average of 26% on 12 occasions, with autoregulation intact 8 times (67%). In one patient, autoregulation was tested on a single occasion at 77 hours post-injury both by increasing and decreasing MABP, with autoregulation found to be intact with both techniques. Thus, there is no obvious difference between raising or decreasing blood pressure in these head-injured patients, so far as changes in CBF and CVR are concerned. Within the first 36 hours post-injury, autoregulation was intact 8 times and defective 7 times. After 36 hours, autoregulation was intact in 13 and defective 7 times (difference not significant). In 9 patients, autoregulation was tested twice. It was intact on both occasions in four, defective twice in one patient, initially intact but later defective in one, and initially defective but later intact in three children. Thus there was no relation between the time post injury at which autoregulation was tested and whether it was intact or not.

Table 4.5 shows the status of autoregulation in relation to the site of injury, as determined by MEP criteria. In all three cases in which the site of injury could not be determined because evoked potentials in all modalities were normal, autoregulation was intact. With purely hemispheric lesions, autoregulation was intact 9 times and defective 8 times. In any case where the brain stem was involved, autoregulation was intact 7 times and defective 5 times. With any diencephalon involvement, it was intact 4 times and defective 2 times. It would thus seem that the site of injury does not determine whether autoregulation will be intact or not.

There was no relation between autoregulation and GCS or outcome. With autoregulation being intact, outcome was favorable 13 times and unfavorable 6 times. With autoregulation defective, outcome was favorable 6 times and unfavorable 6 times (no significant difference).

Table 4.6 shows the relationship between the level of CBF(34) and the status of autoregulation. Autoregulation was relatively more often impaired at the extremes

Table 4.7. Findings in 5 Pediatric Patients in Whom ICP and PVI Could Be Reliably Measured at Two Different Blood Pressures During Tests of Autoregulation*

Case #	Drug	MABP		CBF$_{15}$		ICP		PVI		Autoregulation
		from	to	from	to	from	to	from	to	
129	A	85	70	130	50	10	1	10	16	defective
141	P	100	126	22	30	22	16	9	17	defective
143	P	105	134	39	69	14	20	34	18	defective
148	A	137	90	41	38	26	30	19	17	intact
154	P	103	131	28	41	31	35	23	22	defective

*Drugs: A = Arfonad, P = Phenylephrine. MABP = Mean arterial blood pressure, mmHg. CBF$_{15}$ in ml/100 g/min. ICP in mmHg. PVI in ml.

of the CBF spectrum, i.e., with reduced flow or with absolute hyperemia: intact 5 times and defective 10 times. In the range of normal flows (normal ± 2 SD), autoregulation was intact 15 times and defective 4 times. This difference was statistically highly significant (chi-square = 7.2 1 d.f., p 0.01).

In the 13 cases where autoregulation was tested by raising the blood pressure and found intact, the mean ICP decreased from 17.5 ± 9.2 to 15.0 ± 7.9 mmHg. With intact autoregulation, tested by lowering the blood pressure, mean ICP increased from 20.6 ± 6.9 to 23.4 ± 6.0 mmHg. When autoregulation was defective, ICP increased from 17.1 ± 6.8 to 18.8 ± 7.9 mmHg with higher blood pressure and decreased from 13.3 ± 3.9 to 11.3 ± 8.3 mmHg with lower blood pressure. With autoregulation intact, ICP changed in a direction contrary to what is to be expected 2 out of 21 times; with defective autoregulation, this happened on 4 out of 13 occasions. In a total of 6 cases, ICP did not change with blood pressure changes.

PVI measurements [59] during autoregulation tests were done in 5 children. Results are shown in Table 4.7. In all cases, PVI changed in the opposite direction as the ICP, although in the last 2 cases, these changes were very small. The cases with the largest ICP changes also showed the largest PVI changes. For case 141, one wonders whether autoregulation was indeed defective: during induced hypertension, ICP decreased and PVI increased considerably, indicating vasoconstriction with ensuing diminished CBV which would be more compatible with intact autoregulation. Moreover, AVDO$_2$ remained unchanged (from 6.95 to 6.90), indicating no change in CBF assuming CMRO$_2$ should remain unaltered. Visual inspection of the [133]xenon wash-out curve would indicate that CBF increased and that the calculations of CBF are correct.

There were two children in whom we tried to control ICP by raising the blood pressure. One was an 8-year-old boy, admitted with GCS 7 and a small acute subdural hematoma which was evacuated, whose ICP rose fairly suddenly from 8 to above 25 mmHg 24 hours post injury. This could not be controlled by hyperventilation to a PaCO$_2$ of 19 mmHg, CSF drainage, or mannitol. CBF measurement at that time showed flow of 41 ml/100 g/min bilaterally with AVDO$_2$ of 6.7 vol%. Raising his MABP from 85 to 115 mmHg with phenylephrine brought his ICP down to just below

20 mmHg while his CBF dropped slightly to 38 ml/100 g/min, with $AVDO_2$ of 6.9 vol%. He was kept on phenylephrine for 10 hours, at which time his MABP would spontaneously stay around 100 mmHg with no further ICP problems. He made a good recovery. The other was a 12-year-old boy who was admitted with GCS of 6 and normal CT scan. In the ensuing 5 days he had almost constant ICP problems, which barely could be controlled with CSF drainage, hyperventilation, and mannitol. His PVI hovered around 10 ml, indicating a very stiff brain. On days 4 and 5 post injury, he had received 20 doses of 100 ml of mannitol and when his osmolarity rose above 320, it was decided to induce hypertension as earlier tests of autoregulation had shown a good decrease in ICP with administration of phenylephrine. He was kept on the drug for 3 days, during which time he needed only 5 doses of mannitol, the first of which needed to be given only 24 hours after the initiation of the hypertension therapy. His PVI was around 17 during those days. After 3 days, his blood osmolarity had decreased sufficiently that we preferred to manage ICP further with mannitol alone. Five months later, while recovering but still severely disabled, he died suddenly, presumably from a pulmonary embolus or unwitnessed seizures. Thus, in these two cases where we used induced hypertension to decrease high ICP, this goal was accomplished; but whether this was also clinically beneficial remains completely unproven. We feel that this new type of therapy for increased ICP should be further studied in a limited number of clinical research centers, but its general use certainly cannot be advocated as yet.

One of us has assessed cerebral vascular reactivity to $PaCO_2$ changes [76]. CBF responses assess cerebral vascular regulation to $PaCO_2$ changes. CBF responses to hyperventilation were tested 48 times in 35 patients. The present analysis is based on 31 cases who met the following criteria: one or more tests were administered during the acute illness (less than 96 hours post injury), a physiologically steady state was maintained during the procedure, and the results were not confounded by simultaneous administration of mannitol or barbiturate therapy. Each CO_2 test consisted of two CBF examinations, one during hyperventilation ($PaCO_2$ = 18 to 26 mmHg) and one during a "normoventilation" control condition. Because of intracranial hypertension, however, only a relative degree of normocapnia could be achieved in 15 of the patients ($PaCO_2$ = 28 to 32 mmHg); the remainder had normocapnic CO_2 levels of 34 to 44 mmHg. Order effects were minimized by counterbalancing: hyperventilation preceded the control condition in half of the cases and followed it in the remaining half. From the 31 patients studied, 20 were tested within 24 hours of injury. Seventeen patients were undergoing hyperventilation therapy at the time. Because of intracranial hypertension, some patients were unable to tolerate large $PaCO_2$ increases; nevertheless, a minimal change of 5 mmHg was induced in all occasions. The mean $PaCO_2$ tolerance for the group was 10.6 mmHg, a range of 5 to 20 mmHg. Although 14 patients showed mean arterial pressure changes of 5 to 15 mmHg, there were no systematic blood pressure differences between $PaCO_2$ levels, as the increases balanced the decreases.

Table 4.8. CBF Reactivity to Hyperventilation in Acute Head Injury: Comparison of Two Groups at Different Blood Flow Levels

| CBF Group | Mean and Standard Deviation* | |
	Absolute Reactivity ($\Delta CBF_{15}/\Delta PaCO_2$)	Relative Reactivity (Percent $\Delta CBF_{15}/\Delta PaCO_2$)
Hyperemia (n = 16)	1.4 ± 0.4	3.3 ± 1.1
Reduced flow (n = 13)	0.7 ± 0.3	2.4 ± 0.9

*Absolute, but not relative, reactivity was significantly greater in the hyperemic group (p < 0.002, Mann-Whitney U test).
The symbol Δ denotes changes associated with hyperventilation. ΔCBF_{15} is expressed in ml/100 g/min. The mean $\Delta PaCO_2$ for the sample was 10.6 mmHg.

Both absolute and relative CBF responses to hyperventilation were calculated. Absolute reactivity was defined as CBF change (CBF_{15}/mmHg $PaCO_2$). Relative reactivity, as percent CBF change (ΔCBF divided by CBF_{15}/mmHg $PaCO_2$).

Compared to the normocapnic condition, CBF declined during hyperventilation in 29 patients, all of whom had relative reactivity greater than 1.0%. The remaining two cases showed no response, there being a slight increase in CBF with hyperventilation. Both of these patients underwent neurological decompensation and died within a few days. A decrease in ICP of 3 to 11 mmHg was produced by hyperventilation in 15 cases; the remaining patients showed no change.

In order to determine the effectiveness of hyperventilation at different blood flow levels, CBF responses were compared in two separate groups of patients: those with acute hyperemia and those with reduced flows. Table 4.8 presents such a comparison in the 29 CO_2-reactive cases. One terminal patient in each group was excluded. As shown in Table 4.6, absolute CO_2 reactivity was significantly greater during hyperemia than during reduced flow, confirming the findings of Cold et al [13]. Although there was a trend in the same direction, relative reactivity was not significantly different between groups. For the combined sample, the mean relative reactivity was 2.9%, which compares favorably with normal values reported in the literature. These results indicate that hyperventilation is effective in reducing CBF in acute head injury, especially in patients with hyperemia. Four hyperemic patients retested after 48 hours of prolonged hyperventilation showed no adaptation of the response. The incidence of impaired CO_2 reactivity appears to be low and probably occurs only as a terminal phenomenon. As pointed out in the section on cerebral vascular physiology, a lack of CO_2 reactivity may be the result of a disruption of a blood-brain barrier, indicating a severe primary or secondary insult to the brain and therefore carrying a poor prognosis.

CONCLUDING REMARKS

Results from CBF measurements after severe head injury have been confusing in the past. Data now emerging reveals that the status of the cerebral vasculature can quickly change – especially shortly after the injury – and therefore every attempt must be made to consistently measure CBF early and state exactly (preferably in hours) when the measurements were performed. Furthermore, CBF and cerebral vascular activity may be more important than we had believed in the past, especially since our various forms of therapy all have great impact on CBF and CBV.

Simultaneous measurements of $CMRO_2$ will greatly help us in understanding the underlying pathophysiologic mechanisms, while other adjunctive measurements, such as MEP, may provide data on subtle changes which otherwise could not be assessed. However, there is a definite need for measurements of brain stem blood flow and we need to develop new techniques for this. Our own first experience with stable xenon CT scanning measurements make us hopeful that we can accomplish this goal, but the method is not so easily applicable to patients needing intensive care as the [133]xenon inhalation or intravenous method.

Finally, for those who do not have any method for measuring CBF at their disposal, we would encourage using $AVDO_2$ measurements for monitoring purposes, especially when hyperventilation to very low levels of $PaCO_2$ are used to control ICP.

SUMMARY

In an effort to understand and treat brain pathophysiology resulting from severe head injury, consideration is given to monitoring cerebral blood flow (CBF) and/or cerebral oxygen metabolism ($AVDO_2$, $CMRO_2$). Xenon 133 inhalation or intravenous CBF measurements can be done at the bedside without risk to the patient; but $AVDO_2$ and $CMRO_2$ require a sampling of blood from the right jugular vein. In the future, noninvasive spectroscopy for oxygenation may be able to provide similar information. Measurement of the cerebral perfusion pressure (CPP) reflects perfusion problems related to increased intracranial pressure (ICP) or inadequate mean arterial pressure (MABP) and is a helpful management tool. The relationship of CBF and CPP depends upon cerebral vascular resistance. At present, we do not have a practical method to measure vascular resistance or cerebral blood volume (CBV). A close relationship between an increase in CBV and an increase in ICP exists. However, the relationship between CBF and ICP is more complex. Whereas CBV is strongly dependent upon vasodilation and venous return, CBF is influenced by CPP, vascular resistance, viscosity changes, and focal or diffusely increased ICP. Nevertheless, about two-thirds of patients with increased ICP after head injury have increased CBF (hyperemia) and increased CBV. Thus there is rationale for the wide usage of hyperventilation to treat increased ICP. But it must be recognized that a group of patients may be ischemic due to excessive hyperventilation therapy for ICP. These patients can only be identified by CBF, $AVDO_2$, or similar methods. In such patients, cautiously raising the blood pressure or continuous infusion of mannitol may result in improved CBF, and hyperventilation therapy can be less aggressive.

Conversely, hyperemic patients with increased ICP will usually be improved by further hyperventilation with monitoring of CBF or $AVDO_2$ to avoid ischemia.

The cerebral vasculature, particularly arterioles, are extremely labile but generally react in a predictable fashion (autoregulation) to increased or decreased metabolic demand, blood pressure changes within a physiologic range, viscosity changes, and the $PaCO_2$ content. These alterations may be of critical importance in that a several ml bolus of intracranial volume (i.e., increased CBV, hematoma, contusion, edema, hydrocephalus) can dramatically further increase ICP in a patient with increased ICP and a non-compliant brain. It must be recalled that a diffusely low CBF may well be a byproduct of a comatose state with low metabolism level and not be etiologic. CO_2 and blood pressure reactivity of the cerebral circulation is intact in the majority of head injuries despite common metabolic uncoupling and hyperemia. Autoregulation appears to be more often impaired at the higher or lower extremes of CBF, but a lack of CO_2 reactivity implies a most severe brain insult and blood-brain barrier disruption. The therapeutic utilization of vasoreactivity to improve hyperemia or ischemia and to aid control of ICP, CPP, and brain tissue oxygenation appears to be a realistic goal.

REFERENCES

1. Ackerman RH. The relationship of regional cerebrovascular CO_2 reactivity to blood pressure and regional resting flow. Stroke, 1973, 4:725-731.
2. Adams H, Graham DI. The pathology of blunt head injury. In: Critchley M, O'Leary JL (eds), Scientific Foundations of Neurology. London, W Heinemann, 1972, pp 488-491.
3. Alexander SC, Lassen NA. Cerebral circulatory response to acute brain disease. Anesthesiology, 1970, 32:60-68.
4. Astrup J. Energy-requiring cell functions in the ischemic brain. J Neurosurg, 1982, 56:482-497.
5. Austin G, Horn N, Rouhe S, et al. Description and early results of an intravenous radioisotope technique for measuring regional cerebral blood flow in man. Eur Neurol, 1972, 8:43-51.
6. Bayliss WM. On the local reactions of the arterial wall to changes of internal pressure. J Physiol, 1902, 28:220-231.
7. Brodersen P, Paulson OB, Bolwig TG, et al. Cerebral hyperemia in electrically induced epileptic seizures. Arch Neurol, 1973, 28:334-338.
8. Brown FD, Johns LM, Crockard HA, et al. Response to mannitol following experimental cerebral missile injury. In: Popp AJ, Bourke RS, Nelson LR, et al (eds), Neural Trauma. New York, Raven Press, 1979, pp 281-287.
9. Bruce DA, Alavi A, Bilaniuk L, et al. Diffuse cerebral swelling following head injuries in children: The syndrome of "malignant brain edema." J Neurosurg, 1981, 54:170-178.
10. Bruce DA, Langfitt TW, Miller JD, et al. Regional cerebral blood flow, intracranial pressure, and brain metabolism in comatose patients. J Neurosurg, 1973, 38:131-144.
11. Bruce DA, Raphaely RC, Goldberg AL, et al. Pathophysiology, treatment and outcome following severe head injury in children. Child's Brain, 1979, 5:174-191.
12. Burke AM, Quest DO, Chien S, et al. The effects of mannitol on blood viscosity. J Neurosurg, 1981, 55:550-553.
13. Cold G, Jensen FT, Malmros R. The effects of $PaCO_2$ reduction on regional cerebral blood flow in the acute phase of brain injury. Acta Anesth Scand, 1977, 21:359-367.
14. Craigie EH. The architecture of the cerebral capillary bed. Biol Rev, 1945, 20:133-146.

15. Crockard HA, Brown FD, Trimble J, et al. Somatosensory evoked potentials, cerebral blood flow and metabolism following cerebral missile trauma in monkeys. Surg Neurol, 1977, 7:281-287.

16. Crockard HA, Johns L, Levett J, et al. "Brainstem" effects of experimental cerebral missile injury. In: Popp AJ, Bourke RS, Nelson LR, et al (eds), Neural Trauma. New York, Raven Press, 1979, pp 19-25.

17. DeSalles AAF, Muizelaar JP, Young HF. Hyperglycemia, CSF lactic acidosis and CBF in severely head-injured patients. Neurosurgery, 1987, 21:45-50.

18. DeSalles AAF, Kontos HA, Becker DP, et al. Prognostic significance of ventricular CSF lactic acidosis in severe head injury. J Neurosurg, 1986, 65:615-624.

19. Dieckhoff D, Kanzow E. Uber die Lokalisation des Stromungs-widerstandes in Hirn-kreislauf. Pflugers Arch, 1969, 310:75-85.

20. Ekstrom-Jodal B, Haggendal E, Johannson B, et al. Acute arterial hypertension and the blood-brain barrier: an experimental study in dogs. In: Langfitt TW, McHenry LC Jr, Reivich M, et al (eds), Cerebral Circulation and Metabolism. Berlin, Springer Verlag, 1975.

21. Enevoldsen EM, Cold G, Jensen FT, et al. Dynamic changes in regional CBF, intraventricular pressure, CSF pH and lactate levels during the acute phase of head injury. J Neurosurg, 1976, 44:191-214.

22. Enevoldsen EM, Jensen FT. Autoregulation and CO_2 responses of cerebral blood flow in patients with acute severe head injury. J Neurosurg, 1978, 48:689-703.

23. Fieschi C, Battistini N, Beduschi A, et al. Regional cerebral blood flow and intraventricular pressure in acute head injuries. J Neurol Neurosurg Psychiatry, 1974, 37:1378-1388.

24. Frewen TC, Sumabat WO, Del Maestro RF. Cerebral blood flow, metabolic rate, and cross-brain oxygen consumption in brain injury. J Pediat, 1985, 107:510-513.

25. Fukasawa H. Hemodynamical studies of cerebral arteries by means of mathematical analysis of arterial casts. Tohoku J Exp Med, 1969, 99:255-268.

26. Gee W, Rhodes M, Denstman FJ, et al. Ocular pneumoplethysmography in head-injured patients. J Neurosurgery, 1983, 59:46-50.

27. Gobiet W, Grote W, Bock WJ. The relation between intracranial pressure, mean arterial pressure and cerebral blood flow in patients with severe head injury. Acta Neurochir, 1975, 32:13-34.

28. Graham DI, Adams JH. Ischemic brain damage in fatal head injuries. Lancet, 1971, 1:265-266.

29. Greenberg RP, Newlon PG, Hyatt MS, et al. Prognostic implications of early multimodality evoked potentials in severely head injured patients. A prospective study. J Neurosurg, 1981, 55:227-236.

30. Greenfield JG. The problem of cerebral edema in neurosurgery. Proc R Soc Med, 1947, 40:695.

31. Grubb RL, Raichle ME, Eichling JO, et al. Effects of subarachnoid hemorrhage on cerebral blood volume, blood flow and oxygen utilization in humans. J Neurosurg, 1977, 46:446-453.

32. Haggendal E, Johansson B. Effects of arterial carbon dioxide tension and oxygen saturation on cerebral blood flow and autoregulation in dogs. Acta Physiol Scand, 1965, 66(258):27-53.

33. Halsey JH Jr, Blauenstein UW, Wilson EM, et al. Regional cerebral blood flow comparison of right and left hand movement. Neurology, 1979, 29:21-28.

34. Heistad DD, Marcus ML, Abboud FM. Role of large arteries in regulation of cerebral blood flow in dogs. J Clin Invest, 1978, 62:761-768.

35. Jennett B, Graham DI, Admas H. Ischemic brain damage after fatal blunt head injury. In: McDowell FH, Brennan RW (eds), Cerebral Vascular Disease, Eighth Princeton Conference. New York, Grune and Stratton, 1973, pp 163-170.

36. Jones TH, Morawetz RB, Crowell RM, et al. Threshold of focal cerebral ischemia in awake monkeys. J Neurosurg, 1981, 54:773-782.

37. Kasoff SS, Zingesser LH, Shulman K. Compartment abnormalities of regional cerebral blood flow in children with head trauma. J Neurosurg, 1972, 36:463-470.
38. Kelly PJ, Iwath K, McGraw CP, et al. Intracranial pressure, cerebral blood flow and prognosis in patients with severe head injuries. In: Langfitt TW, McHenry LC Jr, Reivich M, et al (eds), Cerebral Circulation and Metabolism. Berlin, Springer Verlag, 1975, pp 241-244.
39. Kety SS, Schmidt CT. The nitrous oxide method for the quantitative determination of cerebral blood flow in man: theory, procedure and normal values. J Clin Invest, 1948, 27:476-483.
40. Kleinerman J, Sancetta SM. Effect of mild, steady state exercise on general and cerebral hemodynamics of patients with aortic stenosis. J Clin Invest, 1956, 35:717-718.
41. Kontos HA, Raper AJ, Patterson JL Jr. Analysis of vasoactivity of local pH, PCO_2 and bicarbonate on pial vessels. Stroke, 1977, 8:358-360.
42. Kontos HA, Wei EP, Navari RM, et al. Responses of cerebral arteries and arterioles to acute hypotension and hypertension. Am J Physiol, 1978, 234:H371-H383.
43. Kontos HA, Wei EP, Raper AJ, et al. Local mechanism of CO_2 action on cat pial arterioles. Stroke, 1977, 8:226-229.
44. Kontos HA, Wei EP, Raper AJ, et al. Role of tissue hypoxia in local regulation of cerebral microcirculation. Am J Physiol, 1978, 234:H582-H591.
45. Kreutzberg GW, Barron KD, Schubert P. Cytochemical localization of 5'-nucleotidase in glial plasma membranes. Brain Res, 1978, 158:247-257.
46. Kuhn HE, Alavi A, Hoffman EJ, et al. Local cerebral blood volume in head-injured patients, determination by emission computed tomography of ^{99m}Tc-labeled red cells. J Neurosurg, 1980, 52:309-320.
47. Ladurner G, Zilkha E, Sager WD, et al. Measurement of regional cerebral blood volume using EMI 1010 scanner. Br J Radiol, 1979, 52:371-374.
48. Langfitt TW, Obrist WD. Cerebral blood flow and metabolism after intracranial trauma. Prog Neurol Surg, 1981, 10:14-48.
49. Langfitt TW, Obrist WD, Alavi A, et al. Computerized tomography, magnetic resonance imaging and positron emission tomography in the study of brain trauma. Preliminary observations. J Neurosurg, 1986, 64:760-767.
50. Langfitt TW, Tannanbaum HM, Kassell NF. The etiology of acute brain swelling following experimental head injury. J Neurosurg, 1966, 24:47-56.
51. Langfitt TW, Weinstein JD, Kassell NF. Cerebral vasomotor paralysis produced by intracranial hypertension. Neurology, 1965, 15:622-641.
52. Langfitt TW, Weinstein JD, Sklar FH, et al. Contribution of intracranial blood volume to three forms of experimental brain swelling. Johns Hopkins Med J, 1968, 122:261-270.
53. Lassen NA. Cerebral blood flow and oxygen consumption in man. Physiol Rev, 1959, 39:183-238.
54. Lassen NA. The luxury-perfusion syndrome and its possible relation to acute metabolic acidosis localized within the brain. Lancet, 1966, 2:1113-1115.
55. Lassen NA, Ingvar DH. Regional cerebral blood flow measurement in man. Arch Neurol, 1963, 9:615.
56. Laurent JP, Lawner P, Simeone FA, et al. Pentobarbital changes compartmental contribution to cerebral blood flow. J Neurosurg, 1982, 56:504-510.
57. Lou HC, Lassen NA, Friis-Hansen F. Decreased cerebral blood flow after administration of sodium bicarbonate in the distressed newborn infant. Acta Neurol Scand, 1978, 57:239-247.
58. Mangold R, Sokoloff L, Conner E, et al. The effects of sleep and lack of sleep on the cerebral circulation and metabolism of normal young men. J Clin Invest, 1955, 34:1092-1099.
59. Marmarou A, Shulman K, Rosenda RM. A nonlinear analysis of the cerebrospinal fluid system and intracranial pressure dynamics. J Neurosurg, 1978, 48:332-344.

60. Marshall LF, Bruce DA, Bruno L, et al. Vertebrobasilar spasm: a significant cause of neurological deficit in head injury. J Neurosurg, 1978, 48:560-564.
61. Marshall WJS, Jackson JLF, Langfitt TW. Brain swelling caused by trauma and arterial hypertension. Arch Neurol, 1969, 21:545-553.
62. Meyer KL, Dempsey RJ, Roy MW, et al. Somatosensory evoked potentials as a measure of experimental cerebral ischemia. J Neurosurg, 1985, 62:269-275.
63. Miller JD, Garibi J, North JB, et al. Effects of increased arterial pressure on blood flow in the damaged brain. J Neurol Neurosurg Psychiatry, 1975, 38:657-665.
64. Miller JD, Leech HP. Effects of mannitol and steroid therapy on intracranial volume-pressure relationships in patients. J Neurosurg, 1975, 42:274-281.
65. Miller JD, Stanek A, Langfitt TW. Concepts of cerebral perfusion pressure and vascular compression during intracranial hypertension. Progr Brain Res, 1971, 35:411-432.
66. Muizelaar JP, Becker DP. Induced hypertension for the treatment of cerebral ischemia after subarachnoid hemorrhage. Direct effect on cerebral blood flow. Surg Neurol, 1986, 25:317-325.
67. Muizelaar JP, Becker DP, Lutz HA. Present application and future promise of CBF monitoring in head injury. In: Dacey RG, Rimel R, Winn HR, et al (eds), Trauma of the Central Nervous System. New York, Raven Press, 1985, pp 91-102.
68. Muizelaar JP, Becker DP, Lutz HA. Cerebral ischemia after severe head injury: its role in determining clinical status and its possible treatment. In: Villani R, Papo I, Giovanelli M, et al (eds), Advances in Neurotraumatology. Amsterdam, Exerpta Medica, 1983, pp 92-98.
69. Muizelaar JP, Lutz HA, Becker DP. Effect of mannitol on ICP and CBF and correlation with pressure autoregulation in severely head-injured patients. J Neurosurg, 1984, 61:700-706.
70. Muizelaar JP, Obrist WD. Cerebral blood flow and brain metabolism with brain injury. In: Becker DP, Povlishock JD (eds), Central Nervous System Trauma Status Report. Bethesda MD, National Institutes of Health, 1984, pp 123-137.
71. Muizelaar JP, Wei EP, Kontos HA, et al. Mannitol causes compensatory cerebral vasoconstriction and vasodilation in response to blood viscosity changes. J Neurosurg, 1983, 59:822-828.
72. Muizelaar JP, Wei EP, Kontos HA, et al. Cerebral blood flow is regulated by changes in blood pressure and in blood viscosity alike. Stroke, 1986, 17:44-48.
73. Muizelaar JP, Wei EP, Kontos HA, et al. Vasoconstriction with Fluosol-DA as a means of acutely reducing ICP. In: Miller JD, Teasdale GM, Rowan JO, et al (eds), Intracranial Pressure VI. Berlin, Springer Verlag, 1986, pp 758-761.
74. Oberdorster G, Lang R, Zimmer R. Influence of adenosine and lowered cerebral blood flow on the cerebrovascular effects of theophylline. Europ J Pharmacol, 1975, 30:197-204.
75. Obrist WD, Gennarelli TA, Segawa H, et al. Relation of cerebral blood flow to neurological status and outcome in head injured patients. J Neurosurg, 1979, 51:292-300.
76. Obrist WD, Langfitt TW, Jaggi JL, et al. Cerebral blood flow and metabolism in comatose patients with acute head injury. Relationship to intracranial hypertension. J Neurosurg, 1984, 61:241-253.
77. Obrist WD, Thompson HK, Wang HS, et al. Regional cerebral blood flow estimated by 133xenon inhalation. Stroke, 1975, 6:245-256.
78. Obrist WD, Wilkinson WE. The non-invasive Xe-133 method: evaluation of CBF indices. In: Bes A, Geraud G (eds), Cerebral Circulation. Amsterdam-Oxford-Princeton, Exerpta Medica, 1980, pp 119-124.
79. Overgaard J. Tweed WA. Cerebral circulation after head injury. Part 1: Cerebral blood flow and its regulation after closed head injury with emphasis on clinical correlations. J Neurosurg, 1974, 41:531-541.
80. Overgaard J, Tweed WA. Cerebral circulation after head injury. Part 2: The effects of traumatic brain edema. J Neurosurg, 1976, 45:292-299.

81. Overgaard J, Mosdal C, Tweed WA. Cerebral circulation after head injury. Part 3: Does reduced regional cerebral blood flow determine recovery of brain function after blunt head injury? J Neurosurg, 1981, 55:63-74.

82. Pannier JL, Leusen I. Cerebral blood flow in cats after an acute hypertensive insult with damage to the blood-brain barrier. Stroke, 1975, 6:188-198.

83. Perez-Hernandez MJ, Anderson DK. Autoregulation of cerebral blood flow and its relation to cerebrospinal fluid pH. Am J Physiol, 1976, 231:929-935.

84. Pickard JD, MacDonnell A, MacKenzie ET, et al. Response of the cerebral circulation in baboons to changing perfusion pressure after indomethacin. Circ Res, 1977, 40:198-203.

85. Purves MJ. Do vasomotor nerves significantly regulate cerebral blood flow? Circ Res, 1978, 43:485-493.

86. Raichle ME, Grubb RL, Gado MH, et al. Correlation between regional cerebral blood flow and oxidative metabolism. Arch Neurol, 1976, 33:523-526.

87. Raisis JE, Kindt GW, McGillicuddy JE, et al. The effects of primary elevation of cerebral venous pressure on cerebral hemodynamics and intracranial pressure. J Surg Res, 1979, 26:101-107.

88. Reivich M, Marshall WJS, Kassell NF. Loss of autoregulation produced by cerebral trauma. In: Brock M, Fieschi C, Ingvar DH, et al (eds), Cerebral Blood Flow. Berlin, Springer Verlag, 1969.

89. Roquefeuil B, Baldy-Moulinier M, Frerebeau P, et al. Interet de l'exploration metabolique cerebrale dans les etats de coma post-traumatique. Neuro-Chirurgie, 1977, 23:401-412.

90. Rosenblum WI, Zweifach BW. Cerebral microcirculation in the mouse brain. Arch Neurol, 1963, 9:414-423.

91. Rosenstein J, Wang ADJ, Symon L, et al. Relationship between hemispheric cerebral blood flow, central conduction time, and clinical grade in aneurysmal subarachnoid hemorrhage. J Neurosurg, 1985, 62:25-30.

92. Scheinberg P, Stead EA Jr. The cerebral blood flow in male subjects as measured by the nitrous oxide technique. Normal values for blood flow, oxygen utilization, glucose utilization, and peripheral resistance, with observations on the effect of tilting and anxiety. J Clin Invest, 1949, 28:1163-1171.

93. Schrader J, Wahl M, Kuschinsky W, et al. Increase of adenosine content in cerebral cortex in the cat during bicuculline-induced seizure. Pflugers Arch, 1980, 387:245-251.

94. Shapiro HM, Stromberg DD, Lee DR, et al. Dynamic pressures in the pial arterial micro-circulation. Am J Physiol, 1971, 221:279-283.

95. Shigeno T, Brock M, Shigeno S, et al. The determination of brain water content: micro-gravimetry versus drying-weighing method. J Neurosurg, 1982 , 57: 99-108.

96. Sokoloff L, Mangold R, Wechsler RL, et al. The effect of mental arithmetic on cerebral circulation and metabolism. J Clin Invest, 1955, 34:1101-1108.

97. Suwanwela C, Suwanwela N. Intracranial arterial narrowing and spasm in acute head injury. J Neurosurg, 1972, 36:314-323.

98. Symon L. A comparative study of middle cerebral pressure in dogs and macaques. J Physiol, 1967, 191:449-465.

99. Tomita M, Gotoh F, Sato T, et al. Variations in resistance of larger and smaller parts of cerebral arteries with CO_2 inhalation, exsanguination, and vasodilator administration. Acta Neurol Scand, 1977, (Suppl), 64:302-303.

100. Uzell BP, Obrist WD, Dolinskas CA, et al. Relationship of acute CBF and ICP findings to neuropsychological outcome in severe head injury. J Neurosurg 65, 1985, 65:630-635.

101. Wahl M, Deetjen P, Thurau K, et al. Micropuncture evaluation of the importance of perivascular pH for the arteriolar diameter on the brain surface. Pflugers Arch, 1970, 316:152-163.

102. Wahl M, Kuschinsky W. Unimportance of perivascular H+ and K+ activities for the adjustment of pial arterial diameter during changes of arterial blood pressure in cats. Pflugers Arch, 1979, 382:203-208.
103. Wei P, Kontos HA, Patterson JL. Dependence of pial arteriolar response to hypercapnia on vessel size. Am J Physiol, 1980, 238:H697-H702.
104. Winn HR, Rubio R, Berne RM. Brain adenosine concentration during hypoxia in rat. Am J Physiol, 1980, 239(5):H636-H641.
105. Winn HR, Welsh JE, Rubio R, et al. Brain adenosine production in rat during sustained alteration in systemic blood pressure. Am J Physiol, 1980, 239:H636-H641.
106. Wozney P, Yonas H. Latchaw RE, et al. Central herniation revealed by focal decrease in blood flow without elevation of intracranial pressure: a case report. Neurosurgery, 1985, 17:641-644.
107. Yoshino E, Yamaki T, Higuchi T, et al. Acute brain edema in fatal head injury: analysis by dynamic CT scanning. J Neurosurg, 1985, 63:830-839.
108. Zimmerman RS, Muizelaar JP, Wei EP, et al. Acute cerebral arteriolar responses following cold injury. In: Cervos-Navarro J, Terset A (eds), Pathology of the Cerebral Microcirculation. New York, Raven Press, 1987.
109. Zweifach BW. Functional Behavior of the Microcirculation. Springfield, Thomas, 1961.

Chapter 5

Electroencephalography
in Head Injury

James L. Stone, Ramsis F. Ghaly, John R. Hughes,
Albino Bricolo, and Frederic A. Gibbs

Radiologic studies can demonstrate intracranial hemorrhage and structural abnormalities in the injured brain, but only clinical examination or neurophysiological methods can assess the functional integrity of cerebral and brainstem neuronal circuits. Neurophysiological assessment is especially important in comatose patients and may have treatment and prognostic implications. The scalp recorded electroencephalogram (EEG) samples spontaneous cerebral cortical potentials which are influenced by mesencephalic and hemispheric structures. EEG methods have found clinical utility in the evaluation of acute post-traumatic coma and related states of increased intracranial pressure (ICP).

Microvolt or submicrovolt scalp or neck recorded potentials in response to auditory, somatosensory, or visual stimuli are termed sensory evoked potentials (EPs). Recent clinical studies suggest EP correlation with neurological findings in head trauma, lesion localization, intracranial pressure, brain herniation, and prognosis. (See Table 5.1 and Chapter 6.)

The established uses of standard and computerized EEG in acute head injury are outlined in this chapter. Emphasis is placed on EEG correlation with level of consciousness, rostro-caudal deterioration, brainstem lesions, and prognosis. The utility of the standard EEG in seizures and toxic-metabolic states accompanying severe head injury is also discussed.

81

Table 5.1. EEG vs EP

Electroencephalography (EEG)*	Evoked Potentials (EP)**
Definition	
Surface summation of all ongoing electrical brain activity	Surface recorded neurophysiologic response to the appropriate external stimuli that travel from receptor organ along the corresponding neural tract
Activity	
Spontaneous	Externally elicited
Originators	
Cortical (pyramidal) cells	Stimulated sensory neural pathway
Voltage	
> 20 μV	< 20 μV
Signal averaging system	
Not required	Required
Classification	
Frequency	Auditory (AEP), Visual (VEP), Somatosensory (SEP)
Alpha: 8 – 13 Hz	Short (BAEP, SSEP), Middle, Long Latency Potential
Beta: > 13 Hz	Near, Far Field Potential
Theta: 4 – 7 Hz	
Delta: < 4 Hz	

*Chapter 5. **Chapter 6.

STANDARD EEG

The EEG has long been known to show good correlation with a reduced level of consciousness [1,20,26]. High voltage slow wave activity was considered a consequence of increased ICP, somewhat similar to that found in deeper sleep [33,64]. In experimental animals, cerebral concussion was found to be associated with immediate EEG amplitude reduction followed by a short period (seconds to minutes) of slow wave activity, after which the EEG normalized [65]. Similar changes were noted in humans after concussion and follow-up EEG in post-traumatic coma approximates clinical improvement [21,22,23,33].

Experimental and clinicopathologic studies indicated that the ascending reticular activating system, located in man between the lower one-third of the pons and the posterior diencephalon, is essential to arousal [45]. Likewise, the rostral brainstem appears to be essential for alertness and conscious processes by maintaining telencephalic "tonus" [8,44]. A state of unconsciousness or coma following head injury may reflect bilateral hemispheric lesions, a critically located brainstem ascending reticular formation lesion, or both [49]. Behavioral wakefulness (consciousness), EEG arousal (usually desynchronization), and sleep appear to depend on different yet related brainstem reticular and cerebral mechanisms. Most conditions that alter consciousness behaviorally also alter the EEG. However, EEG arousal, sleep potentials, and an alpha rhythm may occur in the presence of impaired consciousness or coma [39,40,49].

Generalized slowing of the EEG after head injury tends to correlate with a depressed level of consciousness, but focal slowing, often temporal in adults and posterior in children, may be transient or permanent. But these EEG abnormalities often have clear diagnostic or surgical significance [37,54,63]. For instance, the EEG of a patient with a significant subdural hematoma could be normal or abnormal on the basis of focal or generalized slow waves and amplitude depression. Consequently, an EEG in acute trauma may poorly localize a clot and lack reliability. Decisions to order diagnostic tests, such as CT scan or angiograms, must be made on the basis of clinical rather than EEG findings [9]. Extracerebral factors, such as scalp edema, subgaleal hemorrhage, or electrode impedance asymmetry, must be excluded before focal depressions or EEG activity can be taken as pathologic [4].

Slowing of the predominant background rhythm has been well delineated and correlated with the clinical findings of a reduced level of consciousness and rostro-caudal deterioration. The mildest grade is found in records with predominantly alpha (8 to 13 Hz) with little intermixed theta (4 to 7 Hz) wave activity; next, a more severe grade includes predominant theta with some delta (1 to 3 Hz); then predominant high voltage rhythmic and arrhythmic delta (1 Hz); and the diffuse delta of low amplitude, appearing only as burst-suppression; and finally electrocerebral silence. With progression, the diffuse slow tends to dominate focal abnormalities [17,19,52].

Other EEG patterns found in acute post-traumatic coma include: superimposed fast activity—frontal predominant or diffuse; normal or altered sleep potentials (spindles, vertex sharps, K-complexes); spontaneous alternating EEG with delta bursts—short (2 to 4 sec) or long (5 sec or longer) duration; lateralizing signs or asymmetries of activity; and reactivity to external stimuli—usually nociceptive or auditory. EEG reactivity may be immediate or delayed and includes desynchronization or attenuation of the EEG pattern, the appearance of widespread delta or theta rhythms, or the appearance of typical or atypical sleep potentials [5,17,19,51,55,59].

Early midbrain dysfunction (drowsiness progressing to coma), as commonly seen in tentorial or uncal herniation, is associated with slight or moderate diffuse slowing which progresses with further dysfunction. Sensory stimulation may briefly block slow wave activity or cause arousal from sleep. Persisting identifiable sleep potentials tend to indicate relatively intact thalamocortical pathways and cortex [8,34,39]. With further clinical midbrain dysfunction (i.e., decerebration and early third nerve findings), a decrease of both spontaneous sleep potentials and alternating patterns generally indicates increasing disturbance of diencephalic and mesencephalic systems. However, stimulation may elicit typical or atypical sleep potentials or a paradoxical arousal with a build-up of diffuse or frontal predominant hypersynchronous delta activity. Later, midbrain and bulbar states secondary to uncal herniation demonstrate more simplified monomorphic delta EEG patterns with absence of both sleep potentials and alternating patterns, suggesting diencephalic damage. Bulbar states show no EEG reactivity, but patients with a central pontine lesion can show EEG desynchronization on passive eye opening [19,30,52,55,59,62].

There is an overall decrease in the number of different EEG patterns relating to the clinical findings of rostral to caudal brainstem dysfunction. This progression has been assumed to indicate increasing ICP, but no specific EEG pattern has been correlated with mean ICP [46,51]. Increasing depth of coma and unfavorable prognosis is associated with loss of sleep potentials, alternating EEG patterns, and EEG reactivity. Conversely, the presence of sleep potentials and reactivity to stimuli is associated more often with recovery [6,11,17,19,48,52].

Bricolo [9] classified patients with acute post-traumatic coma into several fairly distinct EEG groups carrying significantly different survival rates. EEG was recorded as soon as possible after injury and repeated frequently in the following days. Electrocerebral silence was, of course, 100% fatal; and a "monophasic," unorganized, nonreactive polymorphic slow wave record had a mortality of 86%. "Diphasic" records consisted of high amplitude slow waves (spontaneous or evoked) mixed with faster low amplitude background. Mortality was 60%. A "borderline" pattern (7 to 8 Hz) which had similarity to a normal tracing except for a slow background rhythm that was relatively non-reactive to stimuli had a mortality rate of 51%. Diphasic EEG records with "sleep-like" diffuse spindles, variable background, and reactivity consisting of high amplitude rhythmic delta activity showed a mortality of only 13%. The last three patterns indicate the brain is capable of elaborating rhythms and the two diphasic patterns prove the brain can modify its electrical activity spontaneously and/or in an evoked manner [9].

Although a direct brainstem injury may show clinical signs identical to those of a patient with secondary brainstem damage from downward herniation (i.e., decerebration with pupillary dilatation), the EEG could differentiate the two conditions. Patients in coma primarily due to a tegmental brainstem (reticular) lesion, usually pontine or ponto-mesencephalic, may demonstrate diffuse alpha activity ("alpha coma"), at times maximal on the frontal areas [18,30,40,63]. The occasional presence of sleep potentials and EEG reactivity to stimuli in traumatic cases suggests the lesion is below an intact thalamocortical projection system [10]. Later during the first week, these rhythms may be replaced by delta waves [16]. Mortality appears to be greater than 50% in these patients and many survivors remain severely disabled [12,13,62]. Prognosis in coma after head injury is better if the alpha coma represents an additional complication of drug abuse or if spontaneous faster rhythms are slow due to mild diffuse injury complicated by toxic-metabolic encephalopathy [15,47].

Ventral pontine or mesencephalic lesions, including basilar artery thrombosis, may be seen after trauma and tend to produce a "locked-in" or "de-efferented" state. This clinical picture is typified by alertness with mutism, quadriplegia, small pupils, and extraocular movement problems. The patient may be able to communicate with vertical eye movements or eye blinking. The EEG of a "locked-in" patient usually shows more reactive alpha activity than that of a comatose patient [50,62].

Another EEG pattern found within a few days of severe head injury is "spindle coma" consisting basically of normal sleep and spontaneous or evoked sleep potentials [17,32,54]. Spindles at 12 to 14 Hz, sleep-like and often noted beyond the vertex regions, are found in more than half of patients in acute post-traumatic coma. This finding generally carries a good prognosis for survival unless the spindles are asymmetrically distributed or decrease on follow-up tracing. Midbrain involvement with sparing of thalamic structures has been proposed [6,10,11,29,53,59]. The presence of REM sleep during polygraphic recording is more common in lighter coma and also has a favorable prognosis [2,11].

Generalized burst suppression is usually found in post-traumatic coma only when a cerebral anoxic insult has been superimposed [52,59]. The burst suppression activity due to an overdosage of depressant drugs tends to produce a more uniform burst-suppression activity. By contrast, the bursts of activity in anoxic coma are more irregular with delta waves and also intermittent spikes frequently observed [59]. Prognosis is poorer in the latter. A nonreactive alpha coma pattern can also be produced by diffuse anoxia [3,4,53].

COMPUTERIZED EEG

In order to evaluate sleep patterns and electrographic cycling in the days and weeks following injury, the EEG must be recorded frequently and over an extended period of time (preferably at least one continuous 24 hour period). The larger volume of data resulting from long term EEG monitoring and the need for presentation in a more practical format has necessitated the use of computer assisted (Fourier transfer) analysis using compressed spectral array (CSA) or similar techniques. With this method, the power spectra of specific EEG frequency bands may be monitored long-term. The dominant frequencies and their distribution and amplitude may be better assessed with CSA than with conventional EEG. CSA data is readily displayed for easy interpretation. Two or four channels appear to be adequate for CSA evaluation of post-traumatic coma and significant data regarding outcome may be produced [12,13,14,36,57,58] (Figures 5.1 to 5.4).

In one study of 123 comatose (87 head injury) patients, 95% who showed a slow and monotonous CSA had an unfavorable outcome—compared to 30% with a changeable CSA [13]. Using the CSA, worse outcome was also noted among patients with significant interhemispheric amplitude asymmetry [13]. In another study, clinical and CSA examinations were combined to predict outcome in 506 severely head-injured patients with an upper midbrain syndrome. Mortality was 93% if the CSA was slow and monotonous, 57% if borderline, 46% if changeable, and 28% if sleep rhythms were present [12]. Similar results were noted in a study of 100 patients with post-traumatic coma who had CSA examination within 3 days of injury and again within 2 weeks. Mortality was 88% with slow monotonous, 59% with changeable diphasic (delta-alpha), and 13% with changeable sleep-like CSA [57].

The prognostic value of CSA in coma was found to equal that of the neurologic exam and the presence of alternating patterns was significantly associated with survival [36]. In another study of 51 comatose patients (32 head injuries), persistence or return of activity within the alpha or theta range in the first 10 days of coma was

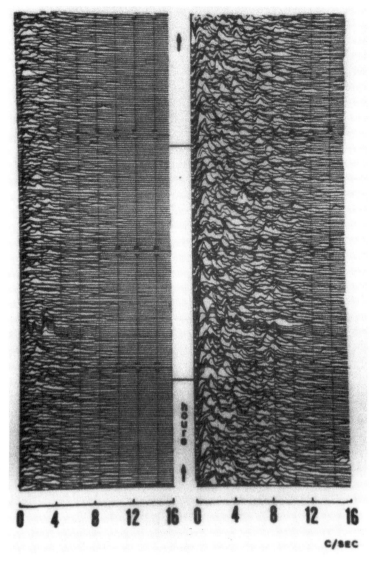

Figure 5.1. Two channel compressed spectral array (CSA) showing interhemispheric asymmetry with diminished power and slower frequencies on the right side (R). The patient had a right sided subdural hematoma previously removed. Central to occipital linkage.

seen in all patients who made a good recovery [14]. In another study, 50 patients with severe brain trauma underwent CSA on the 1st, 2nd, 3rd, 5th, and 7th day after injury. An increase in absolute and relative amplitudes of the alpha and theta ranges correctly predicted survival [58]. In the latter study, several incorrectly predicted cases were of the alpha coma variety or had been given barbiturates for seizures.

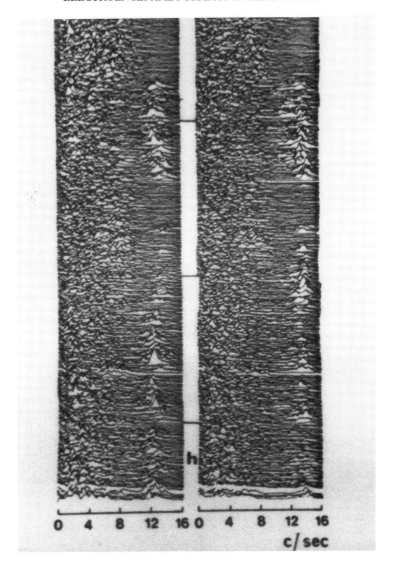

Figure 5.2. Two channel CSA showing a changeable pattern including frequencies within the range of sleep-like activity (12 to 14/sec). The patient had a favorable clinical course after injury. Central to occipital linkage.

STANDARD EEG: SEIZURES AND METABOLIC STATES

The detection and follow-up of seizures and metabolic encephalopathy remains an important use of routine EEG in stuporous or comatose patients. Both seizures and systemic metabolic disturbances are more common in severely injured patients. These secondary insults frequently leave the patient in a deteriorated clinical and

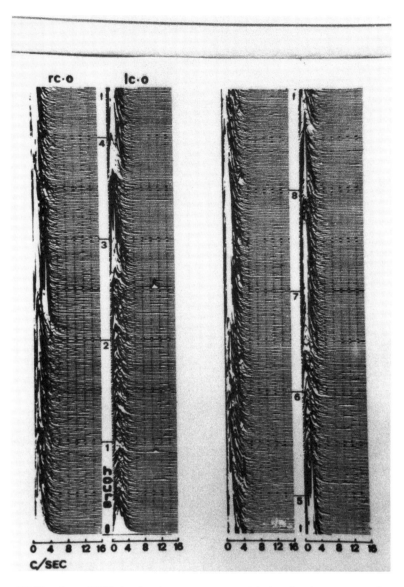

Figure 5.3. Two channel CSA showing slow monotonous activity in a deeply comatose patient with a traumatic mesencephalic syndrome leading to death several days later. Central to occipital linkage.

electrographic state and may lead to permanent structural damage if not promptly corrected. Subclinical seizures could otherwise escape identification and early treatment. Metabolic derangement, drugs, or trauma itself can lower the seizure threshold favoring a focal or generalized seizure [9,51,59].

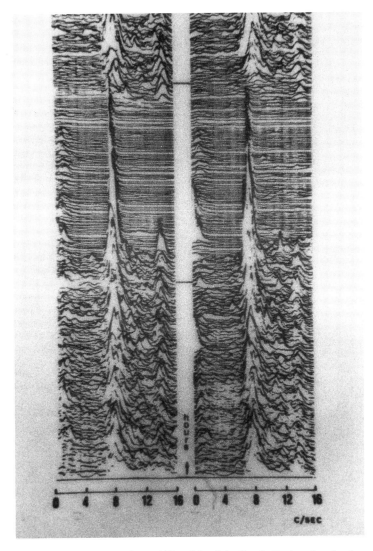

Figure 5.4. Two channel CSA showing stability of the alpha (borderline) peak and a changeable recording including peaks in the sleep-like and delta ranges, in a comatose patient with pontine involvement three days following basilar artery thrombosis. the 8/sec borderline peak was unchangeable and not modified by stimulation for the first several days after injury. This patient survived with severe neurologic impairment. Central to occipital linkage.

Seizures within 1 to 2 weeks of the injury are encountered in roughly 4% of civilian head injuries and 9% of missile head injuries. In a large series, 13% of patients in post-traumatic coma had seizures within this time period, 80% of these within the first five days [9]. Seizures within one week after head injury (early seizures) increase mortality in the adult approximately threefold compared to patients without seizures. Status epilepticus within the first few days after severe head injury carries a mortality over 50% [47,51]. Subclinical, purely electrographic seizures, although uncommon in post-traumatic coma, may precede clinical seizures and imply a worse prognosis [9]. The presence of early seizures also increases the risk for late seizures by approximately fourfold [1,9,35]. Seizure activity and status epilepticus are more common in traumatized children than in adults, but this does not carry a more severe prognosis in children [1,28,56].

Most early post-traumatic seizures are clonic (simple partial) focal motor attacks. The face is often involved and the seizure may progress in Jacksonian fashion to status epilepticus of a hemiclonic or generalized nature [9]. Generalized motor seizures in acute post-traumatic states are less common than focal seizures, and they are usually a consequence of rapid secondary generalization from a lateralized or mesial focus. With focal seizures, the EEG often shows a spike, sharp wave, or spike and wave discharge at 2 to 3 Hz interrupted by suppressed periods. Periodic lateralized epileptiform discharges (PLEDs) are rare after head injury but have been reported with subdural hematoma [60]. Well organized, generalized discharges, such as the 3/sec spike and wave complex, associated with absence, have not been encountered as a result of trauma [1].

It is important to recognize and treat seizures since they may be a cause of hypoxic insult, increased ICP, and secondary brain damage. Generalized seizures are a well established cause of increased cerebral blood flow and volume [25,43]. This results in an increase in ICP that closely follows the spike frequency and electrographic ictal build-up [24]. These changes apply to focal and subclinical seizures and to comatose patients with pharmacologic muscle paralysis or barbiturate coma [24,41,42,61]. The cerebral blood flow and ICP rise during seizure activity does not appear to be dependent on an increase in heart rate or arterial blood pressure [42].

The EEG is influenced by the effects of hypothermia and sedative, anticonvulsant, or anesthetic agents which may obscure both clinical and EEG signs of deterioration. Slowing of the background EEG activity, diffuse slow waves, and frontal predominant fast activity are the most common findings [4,54]. Yet, the frequent use of muscle relaxants, barbiturates, and controlled ventilation as part of intensive care unit control of ICP calls for neurophysiologic methods to monitor central nervous system function.

CONCLUSION

The scalp recorded EEG in head injury provides excellent information about the total amount and severity of brain malfunction, and it is helpful in differentiating direct versus secondary brainstem involvement. Frequent and prolonged EEG recordings in the days immediately following post-traumatic coma can yield information of definite prognostic value. The standard EEG is also valuable in diagnosis, treatment, and follow-up of seizures and toxic and metabolic states. The recent application of more practical, fewer channel, computerized spectral EEG methods has facilitated long-term recordings in post-traumatic coma with strong prognostic value. The deterioration of continuously monitored EEG, in the absence of medication effect or hypothermia, may be an early sign of a structural lesion, ischemia, or metabolic derangement.

REFERENCES

1. Aicardi J. Epilepsy in Children. New York, Raven Press, 1986, pp 77-79, 224-279.
2. Alexandre A, Rubini L, Nertempi P, Farinello C. Sleep alterations during post-traumatic coma as a possible predictor of cognitive defects. Acta Neurochir, 1979, 28(Suppl):188-192.
3. Alving J, Møller M, Sindrup E, Nielsen BL. "Alpha pattern coma" following cerebral anoxia. Electroenceph Clin Neurophysiol, 1979, 47:95-101.
4. Aminoff MJ. Electroencephalography: General principles and clinical applications. In: Aminoff MJ (ed), Electrodiagnosis in Clinical Neurology, 2nd ed. New York, Churchill Livingston, 1986, pp 21-75.
5. Arfel G. Introduction to clinical and EEG studies in coma. In: Remond A, Harner R, Naquet R (eds), Handbook of Electroencephalography and Neurophysiology, Vol 12. Amsterdam, Elsevier, 1975, pp 5-23.
6. Bergamasco B, Bergamini L, Doriguzzi T, Fabiani D. EEG sleep patterns as a prognostic criterion in post-traumatic coma. Electroenceph Clin Neurophysiol, 1968, 24:374-377.
7. Berger H. Uber das Elektrenkephalogramm des Menschen III. Mitteilung. Arch Psychiat Nervenkr 1931, 94:16-60.
8. Bremer F. Some Problems in Neurophysiology. London, Athlone Press, 1953, pp 26-45.
9. Bricolo A. Electroencephalography in neurotraumatology. Clin Electroenceph, 1976, 7:184-197.
10. Bricolo A, Faccioli F, Turazzi S, Pasut ML. EEG and evoked potentials in brainstem traumatic lesions. In: Villani R, Papo I, Giovanelli M, Gaini SM, Tomei G (eds), Advances in Neurotraumatology. Amsterdam, Exerpta Medica, 1983, pp 79-84.
11. Bricolo A, Gentilomo A, Rosadini G, Rossi GF. Long-lasting post-traumatic unconsciousness. A study based on nocturnal EEG and polygraphic recording. Acta Neurol Scand, 1968, 44:512-532..
12. Bricolo A, Turazzi S, Faccioli F. Combined clinical and EEG examination for assessment of severity of acute head injuries. Acta Neurochir, 1979, Suppl, 28:35-39.
13. Bricolo A, Turazzi S, Faccioli F, Odorizzi F, Sciarretta G, Erculiani P. Clinical application of compressed spectral array in long-term EEG monitoring of comatose patients. Electroenceph Clin Neurophysiol, 1978, 45:211-225.
14. Cant BR, Shaw NA. Monitoring by compressed spectral array in prolonged coma. Neurology, 1984, 34:35-39.
15. Carroll WM, Mastaglia FL. Alpha and beta coma in drug intoxication uncomplicated by cerebral hypoxia. Electroenceph Clin Neurophysiol, 1979, 46:95-105.
16. Chatrian GE. Electroencephalographic and behavioral signs of sleep in comatose states. In: Remond A, Harner R, Naquet R (eds), Handbook of Electroencephalography and Neurophysiology, Vol 12. Amsterdam, Elsevier, 1975, pp 63-77.
17. Chatrian GE, White LE, Daly D. Electroencephalographic patterns resembling those of sleep in certain comatose states after head injury. Electroenceph Clin Neurophysiol, 1963, 15:272-280.

18. Chatrian GE, White LE, Shaw CM. EEG pattern resembling wakefulness in unresponsive decerebrate state following traumatic brain stem infarct. Electroenceph Clin Neurophysiol, 1964, 16:285-289.

19. Courjon J, Scherzer E. Traumatic disorders. In: Remond A, Magnus O, Courjon J (eds), Handbook of Electroencephalography and Neurophysiology, Vol 14. Amsterdam, Elsevier, 1972, pp 3-104.

20. Davis H, Davis PA. The electrical activity of brain. Its relation to physiological states and to states of impaired consciousness. Res Publ Ass Res Nerv Ment Dis, 1939, 19:50-80.

21. Dawson RE, Webster JE, Gurdjian ES. Serial electroencephalography in acute head injuries. J Neurosurg, 1951, 8:613-630.

22. Denny-Brown D, Russell WR. Experimental cerebral concussion. Brain, 1941, 64:93-164.

23. Dow RS, Ulett G, Raaf J. Electroencephalographic studies immediately following head injury. Am J Psychiat, 1944, 101:174-183.

24. Gabor AJ, Brooks AG, Scobey RP, Parsons GH. Intracranial pressure during epileptic seizures. Electroenceph Clin Neurophysiol, 1984, 57:497-506.

25. Gibbs FA, Lennox WG, Gibbs EL. Cerebral blood flow preceding and accompanying epileptic seizures in man. Arch Neurol Psychiat, 1934, 32:257-272.

26. Gibbs FA, Davis H, Lennox WG. The electroencephalogram in epilepsy and in conditions of impaired consciousness. Arch Neurol Psychiat, 1935, 34:1133-1148.

27. Gloor P. Hans Berger on the electroencephalogram of man. Electroenceph Clin Neurophysiol, 1969, Suppl, 28:95-132.

28. Grand W. The significance of post-traumatic status epilepticus in childhood. J Neurol Neurosurg Psych, 1974, 37:178-180.

29. Hansotia P, Gottschalk P, Green P, Zais D. Spindle coma: incidence, clinicopathologic correlates and prognostic value. Neurology, 1981, 31:83-87.

30. Hughes JR, Cayaffa JJ, Leestma J, Mizuno Y. Alternating "waking" and "sleep" EEG patterns in a deeply comatose patient. Clin Electroenceph, 1972, 3:86-93.

31. Hughes JR, Boshes B, Leestma J. Electroclinical and pathologic correlations in comatose patients. Clin Electroenceph, 1976, 7:13-30.

32. Jankel WR, Niedermeyer E. Sleep spindles. J Clin Neurophysiol, 1985, 2:1-35.

33. Jasper HH, Kershman J, Elvidge A. Electroencephalographic studies of injury to the head. Arch Neurol Psychiat, 1940, 44:328-348.

34. Jasper HH, VanBuren J. Interrelationships between cortex and subcortical structures. Clinical EEG studies. Electroenceph Clin Neurophysiol, 1953, Suppl, 4:168-188.

35. Jennett B, Van de Sande J. EEG prediction of post-traumatic epilepsy. Epilepsia, 1975, 16:251-256.

36. Karnaze DS, Marshall LF, Bickford RG. EEG monitoring of clinical coma: The compressed spectral array. Neurology, 1982, 32:289-292.

37. Kiloh LG, Osselton JW. Clinical Electroencephalography. London, Butterworth, 1976, pp 125-138.

38. Krüger J, Steudel WI, Grau HC. Traumatic lesions of the brain stem: Electroencephalographic and computer-tomographic follow-up study in the acute phase. Electroenceph Clin Neurophysiol, 1981, 51:526-536.

39. Lindsley DB, Bowden JW, Magoun HW. Effect upon the EEG of acute injury to the brain stem activating system. Electroenceph Clin Neurophysiol, 1949, 1:475-486.

40. Loeb C, Poggio G. EEG in a case with pontomesencephalic hemorrhage. Electroenceph Clin Neurophysiol, 1953, 5:295-296.

41. Marienne JP, Robert G, Bagnat E. Post-traumatic acute rise of ICP related to subclinical epileptic seizures. Acta Neurochir, 1979, Suppl, 28:89-92.

42. Matsuda M, Nakasu S, Handa J. Intracranial pressure responses to electroencephalographic changes in epileptic seizures and barbiturate coma therapy. In: Ishii S, Nagai H, Brock M (eds), Intracranial Pressure V. Berlin, Springer Verlag, 1983, pp 793-796.

43. Meyer JS, Gotoh F, Favale E. Cerebral metabolism during epileptic seizures in man. Electroenceph Clin Neurophysiol, 1966, 21:10-22.

44. Moruzzi G. Influence of brain stem reticular formation on cortical electrical activity. Electroenceph Clin Neurophysiol, 1949, 1:519.

45. Moruzzi G, Magoun HW. Brainstem reticular function and activation of the EEG. Electroenceph Clin Neurophysiol, 1949, 1:455-473.

46. Munari C, Calbucci F. Correlations between intracranial pressure and EEG during coma and sleep. Electroenceph Clin Neurophysiol, 1981, 51:170-176.

47. Oken BS, Chiappa KH. Electroencephalography and evoked potentials in head trauma. In: Becker DP, Povlishock JT (eds), Central Nervous System Trauma Status Report. Washington, National Institutes of Health, NINCDS, 1985, pp 177-185.

48. Pfurtscheller G, Schwarz G, List W. Long-lasting EEG reactions in comatose patients after repetitive stimulation. Electroenceph Clin Neurophysiol, 1986, 64:402-410.

49. Plum F, Posner JB. The Diagnosis of Stupor and Coma, 2nd ed. Philadelphia, FA Davis, 1972, pp 1-61.

50. Plum F, Posner JB. The Diagnosis of Stupor and Coma, 3rd ed. Philadelphia, FA Davis, 1982, pp 70-72.

51. Rumpl E. Cranio-cerebral trauma. In: Niedermeyer E, Lopes da Silva F (eds), Electroencephalography: Basic Principles, Clinical Applications and Related Fields. Baltimore, Urban & Schwarzenberg, 1982, pp 291-304.

52. Rumpl E, Lorenzi E, Hackl JM, Gerstenbrand F, Hengl W. The EEG at different stages of acute secondary traumatic midbrain and bulbar brain syndromes. Electroenceph Clin Neurophysiol, 1979, 46:487-497.

53. Rumpl E, Prugger M, Bauer G, Gerstenbrand F, Hackl JM, Pallua A. Incidence and prognostic value of spindles in post-traumatic coma. Electroenceph Clin Neurophysiol, 1983, 56:420-429.

54. Saunders MG, Westmoreland BF. The EEG in evaluation of disorders affecting the brain diffusely. In: Klass DW, Daly DD (eds), Current Practice of Clinical Electroencephalography. New York, Raven Press, 1979, pp 343-379.

55. Schwartz MS, Scott DF. Pathological stimulus-related slow wave arousal responses in the EEG. Acta Neurol Scand, 1978, 57:300-304.

56. Silverman D. Electroencephalographic study of acute head injury in children. Neurology, 1962, 12:273-281.

57. Sironi VA, Ravagnati L, Signoroni G, Sganzerla E, Pampini P, Ducati A, Tomei G, Oriani M, Granata G. Diagnostic and prognostic value of EEG compressed spectral analysis in post-traumatic coma. In: Villani R, Papo I, Giovanelli M, Gaini SM, Tomei G (eds), Advances in Neurotraumatology. Amsterdam, Exerpta Medica, 1983, pp 328-330.

58. Steudel WI, Krüger J. Using the spectral analysis of the EEG for prognosis of severe brain injuries in the first post-traumatic week. Acta Neurochir, 1979, Suppl, 28:40-42.

59. Stockard JJ, Bickford RG, Aung MH. The electroencephalogram in traumatic brain injury. In: Vinken PJ, Bruyn GW (eds), Handbook of Clinical Neurology, Vol 23, I. Amsterdam, North-Holland, 1975, pp 317-367.

60. Toyonaga K, Schlagenhauff RE, Smith BH. Periodic lateralized epileptiform discharges in subdural hematoma. Clin Electroenceph, 1974, 5:113-118.

61. Tsementzis SA, Gillingham FJ, Hitchcock ER. The effect of focal twitching on the intracranial pressure during paralysis and mechanical ventilation. Ann Clin Res, 1979, 11:253-257.

62. Turazzi S, Bricolo A. Acute pontine syndromes following head injury. Lancet, 1977, ii:62-64.

63. Westmoreland BF, Klass DW, Sharbrough FW, Reagan TJ. "Alpha coma": EEG, clinical, pathologic and etiologic correlations. Arch Neurol, 1975, 32:713-718.
64. Williams D. The electro-encephalogram in acute head injuries. J Neurol Psychiat, 1941, 4:107-130.
65. Williams D, Denny-Brown D. Cerebral electrical changes in experimental concussion. Brain, 1941, 64:223-238.

Chapter 6

Sensory Evoked Potentials in Head Injury

James L. Stone, Ramsis F. Ghaly, John R. Hughes, and Seigo Nagao

INTRODUCTION

Sensory evoked potentials (EPs) represent neurophysiological responses of sensory pathways to appropriate sensory stimuli. These potentials are often of submicrovolt ($< 10^{-6}$V) amplitude, yet due to advances in electronics and computer averaging, they are readily recorded from the scalp using surface electrodes. EPs can be classified according to the type of stimulation into somatosensory (SEP), auditory (AEP), and visual (VEP) evoked potentials. Recent studies in patients with acute head trauma suggest EP correlation with neurological findings, lesion localization, intracranial pressure, brain herniation, and prognosis.

SEPs are elicited by electrical stimulation of a mixed peripheral nerve, such as the median nerve at the wrist, posterior tibial nerve at the ankle, or peroneal nerve at the knee. Recording electrodes are usually placed over the proximal peripheral nerve or plexus, spinal regions, and somatosensory scalp. Acoustic stimuli (usually broadband click stimuli) delivered to the ear are used for AEP testing with recording electrodes at the vertex (Cz) and ipsilateral ear lobe. For VEP testing, flash, goggles or checkerboard (pattern-shift) stimulation is performed and surface pick-up electrodes placed over the occipital areas. However, pattern-shift VEPs (PSVEP) are more often used because they are more sensitive and reproducible than flash-VEPs, but do require patient cooperation [10,11,34,64,86].

95

Table 6.1. Far- vs. Near-Field EPs

	Far-Field	Near-Field
Origin	Subcortical	Cortical
Transmission	Volume Conduction	Neural Pathway
Latency	Early	Late
Amplitude	Low $< 1\,\mu V$	Large $1-50\,\mu V$
Distribution	Non-Specific Broad Topography	More Specific
Waveform Consistency	Stable	Less Stable
Subject and Psychological Variation	Consistent	Non Consistent
Pharmacological Agents	Less Susceptible	More Susceptible
Uses	Widely Used	Less Used

Sensory evoked potentials are also classified by time of occurrence after stimulation into short, middle, and long latency potentials. Short latency sensory evoked potentials reflect the passage of a response to a specific afferent sensory stimulus generated in the peripheral ascending system or brainstem, and monitor the functional integrity of these two sites. These potentials are also called far-field potentials because the site of scalp recording may be well away from the location of their generators. Short latency potentials also include cochlear and brainstem (< 10 to 15 msec) auditory evoked potentials, and short latency somatosensory evoked potentials (SSEPs) (< 25 to 50 msec, according to the nerve being stimulated). On the other hand, middle and long latency potentials are considered as cortically generated and they are called near-field potentials. Long latency sensory EPs provide evidence for hemispheric function (Table 6.1.).

The electrocochleogram (ECochG) reflects the electrical response of the cochlea and the auditory nerve to acoustic stimulation. Brainstem auditory evoked potentials (BAEP) consist of seven or eight sequential positive peaks following stimulation and labeled by Roman numerals I through VII (Figure 6.1) [65,66,81,95,100,191]. SSEP in response to median nerve stimulation consists of at least six distinct waves with specific polarity (positive [P] or negative [N] polarity) and peak latencies in milliseconds (N_9, N_{11}, N_{13}, P_{14}, N_{20}, P_{23} in Figures 6.2 and 6.3) [9,34,35,38].

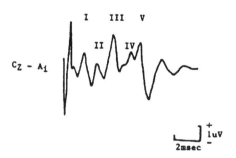

Figure 6.1. Brainstem auditory evoked potentials (BAEPs). Human.

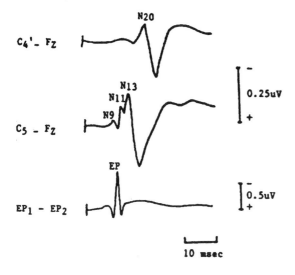

Figure 6.2. Short-latency somatosensory evoked potentials (SSEPs) following unilateral median nerve stimulation at the wrist. Human.

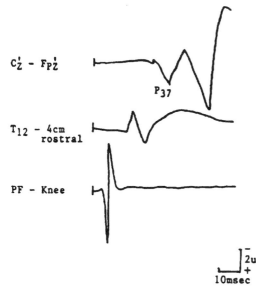

Figure 6.3. Short-latency somatosensory evoked potentials (SSEPs) following unilateral posterior tibial nerve stimulation at the ankle. Human.

Pattern-shift (reversal) VEPs typically (in the first 250 msec) show waves N_{75}, P_{100}, N_{145}, of which P_{100} is considered the most important component (Figure 6.4). In flash-VEP, a sequence of six alternating P and N waves are seen with a prominent positive peak around 100 msec (Figure 6.5) [10,11,32,87].

The possible generator sources of BAEPs and SSEPs are listed in Tables 6.2 and 6.3. Less is known concerning the exact origin of middle and long latency potentials, often believed to reflect thalamo-cortical projections, primary or secondary cortical

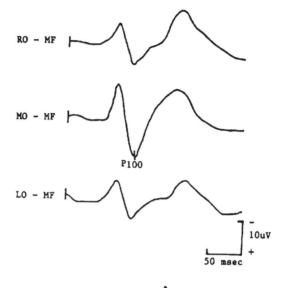

RO – MF

MO – MF

P100

LO – MF

10uV

50 msec

Figure 6.4. Pattern shift (reversal) visual evoked potentials (PSVEPs). Human.

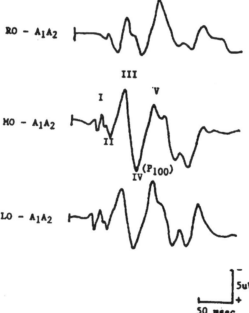

RO – A_1A_2

III

I   V

MO – A_1A_2

II

IV (P_{100})

LO – A_1A_2

5uV

50 msec

Figure 6.5. Flash visual evoked potentials (FVEPs). Human.

association areas. VEPs are generated in the occipital cortex and their components are thought to reflect electrical activity of the visual system [32,33,44,86,143].

Short latency potentials are very resistant to environmental or subject variations whereas middle and long latency potentials show larger inter- and intra-subject

Table 6.2. Possible Generator Sources of BAEP Components Following Auditory
Stimulation in Man

BAEP Component	Generator Source	Level
I	Auditory Nerve	Cochlea-Pontomedullary Entry
II	Auditory Nerve/Cochlear Nucleus	Ponto medullary
III	Olivary Complex	Caudal Pontine
IV	Lateral Lemniscus	Rostral Pontine – Midbrain
V	Inferior Colliculus	Midbrain
VI	Medial Geniculate Body	Thalamic
VII	Thalamocortical Radiation	Thalamic/Thalamocortical

variability. The latter potentials are affected by state of consciousness or attentiveness of the subject, sedatives, barbiturates, and anesthetic agents [94,200]. As a consequence, short latency potentials are more stable and have been more widely used in the intensive clinical setting with critically ill head injury patients.

Latency, interpeak latency (IPL), amplitude, amplitude ratio, interhemispheric difference, and waveform morphology constitute the most common measures used to interpret evoked potentials. In order to determine "normals" or "abnormals," a control sample from the normal population (at least 20 subjects) is recommended for each laboratory using its own equipment. Values beyond 2, 2.5, or preferably 3 standard deviations of the mean or a normal control group are considered abnormal in most laboratories. Generally, isolated amplitude and morphologic changes are not considered criteria of clinically significant abnormality, particularly when absolute latency or IPL is normal [10,11]. There is wide variability in the amplitude of peaks among health subjects. Nevertheless, amplitude measurements may be a sensitive criteria and a good indicator for early dysfunction [198]. For example, amplitude depression of the SEP was a sensitive indicator for reduction of cerebral blood flow (CBF) in stroke patients while latency change was not [120]. A relative amplitude measure such as wave V compared to wave I of the BAEP (normal V/I ratio is greater than 1, abnormality < 0.5) may be useful [198].

Latencies of the different peaks, on the other hand, and interpeak latencies of the BAEP are more consistent and stable than amplitudes in each individual under

Table 6.3. Possible Generator Sources of SEP Components
Following Median and Posterior Tibial Nerve Stimulation in Man

	SEP Component		
	Median	Tibial	Generator Source/Level
P/N	9		Brachial plexus
	11	18-20	Spinal cord entry
	13	27	Dorsal column/dorsal column nuclei
	14	30	Medial lemniscus/brainstem
	18	32	Thalamus/thalamo-cortical radiations
	22	36-38	Parietal somatosensory cortex

normal conditions [41,42,192]. Latency and IPL changes may indicate more serious damage than amplitude changes [10,11].

The N_{13} component after median nerve stimulation at the wrist appears to originate from the brainstem, possibly the dorsal column nuclei. The N_{18-20} component may originate from specific thalamo-cortical projections or somatosensory cortex, whereas the P_{23} component is more clearly of cortical origin [35,36,38]. I-V IPL and $N_{13}/N_{14}-N_{20}$ reflect brainstem auditory or somatosensory central transmission time (CTT). IPL prolongation indicates pathologic dysfunction of the central auditory or somatosensory systems and is considered a sensitive criterion for central (but not peripheral) conduction changes [30,34,36,53,98,196,202].

Delay in latency may indicate slowed conduction, whereas low amplitude may indicate a decrease in the number of active neurons or possibly a change in the extracerebral resistance to recording the signals [198]. Asynchrony of bilateral conduction may cause a variable decrease in amplitude, increase in latency, and waveform distortion. Pathologic insults affecting a conducting neuronal pathway such as disruption, ischemia, or distortion/compression may alter or obliterate EPs [75,146].

Until recently there has been inconsistency in stimulating and recording parameters, and the criteria used to interpret evoked potential abnormalities. For example, differences in filter settings can result in marked differences in the latencies and amplitudes of various waveforms. In the last few years, guidelines for the recording and clinical reporting of evoked potentials have been set forth [10,11].

Integrity of peripheral sensory function should be assessed (when possible) before considering the EP results [34,196]. This assessment is generally performed by recording early components and verifying the adequacy of the sensory input. For example, appropriate ophthalmological examination and electro-retinal testing is recommended in VEP testing. When recording BAEP, peripheral hearing should ideally be verified with an audiogram. Middle ear impedance and pressure abnormalities may be found in comatose head-injured patients and confuse the interpretation of BAEP findings, especially if absolute latency, rather than IPLs, are considered [80,81]. External or middle ear conductive hearing losses are perceived as a decreased stimulus intensity and post-traumatic hemotympanum may complicate BAEP testing in head trauma. In SEP monitoring, slow peripheral nerve conduction velocities due to peripheral nerve injury, relatively long arm or leg length, or hypothermia may account for increased absolute latencies of SEP peaks [34].

To enhance yield of information and display of EPs, serial recording with multi-channel electrode arrays may be used to improve the visualization of certain peaks and verify multiple afferent pathways. Serial EP recording is essential for early detection of insults and for demonstrating progression or regression of EP abnormalities. Repeated testing may be important for timely medical management as well as to monitor the effectiveness of treatment [80,81]. Furthermore, measurement of latency-intensity and amplitude-intensity (input-output functions) of waves I, III, and

V of BAEP at multiple intensities can enhance the utility of BAEP in neurological patients [41,42,63,204]. An increase in stimulation rate may also increase the power of BAEP and VEP testing [41,42,63,163,164,204].

Second to the clinical examination, continuous electrophysiological monitoring has been advocated in intensive care settings as the best available assessment of brain function. Application of sensory EP in the neurotrauma intensive care unit has shown remarkable progress in the past few years. EP monitoring is a safe, noninvasive technique readily performed at the bedside. In a situation where adequate communication with the patient is impossible, EP recording may provide significant functional information that would not be known otherwise. EP recording has been shown to be efficacious in the pediatric as well as adult head-injured population [80,93,158,195].

Evoked potentials have commonly been used not only as a diagnostic test but also as a prognostic indicator. As mentioned above, EPs provide accurate information regarding the functional integrity of the peripheral sensory system, brainstem, and hemispheric functions. Furthermore, changes in arterial oxygenation (PaO2) and carbon dioxide (PaCO2) content, intracranial pressure (ICP), cerebral blood flow (CBF), cerebral perfusion pressure (CPP), and hypothermia may alter or obliterate EPs [39,60,68,108,120,131,135,148,151,194,207]. Metabolic or systemic changes need to be extreme to markedly alter the short latency EPs. The presumption is that early detection and correction of systemic or focal brain insults may improve the morbidity and mortality of head-injured patients. Prompt discovery of abnormal neuronal conducting systems could lead to timely diagnosis and treatment before irreversible damage takes place. Clinico-pathological correlates and the prognostic power of sensory EPs in head injury will be discussed below.

CLINICAL FINDINGS

An abnormal BAEP in comatose head-injured patients may indicate injury to the peripheral auditory apparatus (hemotympanum), eustachian tube dysfunction, middle ear pressure changes, temporal bone fracture or brainstem abnormality [70,71,80,81].

BAEP results and otologic findings were poorly correlated in acute head-injured patients [3]. Otologic disorders were reported in one half of head trauma patients with a normal BAEP. By contrast, an abnormal BAEP due to brainstem insult can be seen in patients with normal otologic examinations [3]. Furthermore, no correlation was found between CT scan findings and BAEP results. A temporal bone fracture could result in a loss of all BAEP waves beyond I or II. A combination of auditory evoked potential assessment, otologic examination, and CT scanning was considered to provide complementary information about the functional or structural status of the peripheral and central auditory system. Auditory follow-up and temporal bone CT analysis was recommended in patients with both an abnormal BAEP and otologic examination [3].

Although there is no linear correlation between the Glasgow Coma Scale (GCS) [208] and evoked potential findings, a higher incidence of evoked potential abnormalities occurred in patients with a low GCS score [84,126,130]. Patients with a GCS of 8 or less are considered to have a severe head injury; and GCS of 9 to 13, a more moderate injury. In a study of 111 traumatically head-injured patients, 52% of 95 patients with GCS of 3 or 4 had an abnormal BAEP recording—in contrast to only 19% of the 16 patients with GCS of 7 or greater [130]. Evoked potentials reflect sensory phenomena, whereas GCS includes important prognostic motor functions. Nevertheless, the optimal motor response of GCS was found to correlate with SEP and VEP, but not with BAEP and AEP. The overall coma score provided a similar correlation [125,126]. Another study showed good agreement between a normal BAEP and a GCS above 7, and also between an abnormal BAEP and a GCS below 5. There was no correlation between BAEP changes and a GCS of 5 to 7, although BAEP predicted outcome in this group with an accuracy rate of 81% [25].

Normal BAEP has been reported in patients with severe neurological dysfunction, including the brainstem [84,85]. Normalization of an abnormal BAEP was a good indicator for clinical improvement and a deterioration of the BAEP was seen in patients with clinical neurological deterioration [150]. Persistent EP abnormalities were seen in patients likely to remain severely disabled [142].

Brainstem dysfunction can be assumed when short latency auditory and somatosensory evoked potentials are present but severely abnormal. On the other hand, hemispheric dysfunction can be expected in patients with severely abnormal or absent VEP (long latency), SEP and/or AEP [188]. The duration of coma, decerebration, and decortication were correlated with cerebral hemispheric dysfunction detected by cortical and subcortical (far-field) EPs [70,71]. Good agreement was present between intact brainstem reflexes and a normal BAEP, but not between an abnormal BAEP and brainstem reflexes [25].

Decerebration was associated with BAEP abnormalities including increased latency of all components and instability of the peaks. Recovery of these abnormalities was recorded later than recovery from decerebration [113]. However, decerebrate patients may show normal BAEP, suggesting that posturing may relate to hemispheric and not brainstem dysfunction [71,106,213].

Absence of BAEP components, except wave I, was a common finding in flaccid patients, whereas a normal BAEP recording was more often found in patients with flexion reactivity [213]. The majority of patients with bilateral dilated and fixed pupils showed abnormalities in (or absence of) wave V, IV, and III. Preservation of wave V correlated well with intact vertical eye movements, while preservation of wave III was correlated with intact horizontal eye movements. Unilateral pupillary abnormalities were associated with abnormalities in wave IV and V, or normal BAEP [126,213].

A significant association was found between the BAEP and oculo-cephalic reflex in that an absence of the oculo-cephalic reflex for 8 hours was associated with absence of the peaks beyond wave I [107]. Another study showed no relation among BAEP abnormalities, corneal reflex and posturing abnormalities [57].

BAEP changes were found to correlate with the clinical findings of transtentorial herniation and brainstem compression [57,132,148,150,212]. Furthermore, in that setting, BAEP changes were recorded earlier than clinical changes [4,25,132,144,212]. Changes in wave V amplitude was well correlated with pupillary signs during herniation, which appears to reflect marked ischemia of the upper brainstem associated with uncal herniation in the cat [144,151] and monkey [205]. BAEP changes can be seen in patients with brainstem ischemia before the onset of clinical deterioration. BAEP changes also may correlate with clinical signs of increased ICP [19,20,152]. Wave III was found to be a sensitive indicator for medullary failure and respiratory arrest [152]. Normalization of wave V latency was seen following the use of IV hypertonic solution in patients with high ICP due to supratentorial mass lesions. However, pupillary normalization was only seen in a limited number of patients [144].

Intact pupillary responses and oculo-vestibular reflexes were associated with preservation of long and middle latency auditory potentials [180]. Absence of long latency potentials with intact middle latency potentials did not correlate with normal pupillary and oculo-vestibular responses [180]. The presence of cranial nerve reflexes was associated with intact VEP and SEP whereas absence of cranial nerve reflexes were associated with lost SEP and VEP [210].

SEP changes can also be seen with cerebral ischemia and hypoxia [130,207]. Good agreement was observed between cortical activation produced either by peripheral nerve stimulation or voluntary movement and regional cerebral blood flow [60]. Recovery of evoked response was seen after correction of the causative vascular insult or systemic hypoxia [24,75,120]. SEP abnormalities were reported in trauma patients with hemiparesis or hemiplegia and the chance of recovery was predicted from the severity of SEP abnormalities [12,71,126]. Persistent asymmetry of the SEP was also reported in hemiplegic brain-injured patients [12,71,98]. Multimodality evoked potentials (MEPs) were found useful in detecting regional or global dysfunction in trauma patients [71,188].

Sensory EPs may successfully be used to assess patients under conditions in which neurological examination and other investigations may be misleading. For example, BAEP is a valuable test to assess patients in barbiturate coma at a time when EEG and neurological examinations are severely altered. Related conditions include chemically paralysed patients and patients sedated to control respirations and intracranial pressure.

Evoked potentials are less helpful regarding etiology of the lesion or pathologic process. However, sensory EPs can provide some diagnostic clues and substantiate a suspicion of an intrinsic brainstem lesion or impending herniation. BAEP was

Table 6.4. Criteria Used for Studying Sensory Evoked Potentials

Absolute latency
Interpeak latency (IPL) — Central conduction time (CCT)
Amplitude and amplitude ratio
Interhemispheric latency and amplitude difference
Waveform morphology

reported to be of diagnostic importance in differentiating comatose patients with brainstem lesions from those with metabolic or psychogenic disorders [91,191,201,202]. BAEP is expected to be abnormal if the underlying etiology of coma is a sizable brainstem lesion, but more likely normal if the underlying etiology is metabolic or psychogenic [131,201,202].

Serial recordings have been recommended by many investigators to assess the patient's condition throughout the critical medical period and to provide an accurate evaluation of brain function at the time of recording. Delayed systemic or intracranial insults are common in severe head-injured patients and serial recordings may be helpful [70,125,131,154,156,166,212]. At some point in the future, sensory EPs may become an even more effective guide in the treatment of post-traumatic coma.

Cortical and subcortical evoked potentials can correlate with post-traumatic findings such as cognitive impairment, post-concussion syndrome, and behavioral disorders [20,72,76,119,157,162,163,168,175]. Fifty-five patients with post-concussion syndrome underwent BAEP testing [19] and 15 showed abnormal responses, particularly prolonged IPLs, while nine had borderline abnormal responses. No correlation was found between BAEP changes and dizziness or caloric vestibular dysfunction. However, there was a good agreement between BAEP improvement and recovery of the post-concussion syndrome [19].

A conclusion that P_{300} latency of auditory evoked potential was the most sensitive indicator of traumatic brain dysfunction was made in a study of 18 head trauma patients [162]. A strong correlation was found between P_{300} latency and neuropsychological measures, especially with those for orientation and memory. A return to normal values was associated with recovery of cognitive impairment. In another study P_{300} latency was thought to correlate with post-traumatic amnesia (PTA) and normalized with the resolution of PTA [167].

The VEP was felt to be a sensitive indicator for post-traumatic cognitive and interactive behavioral dysfunction [76,157,164,175]. The severity of cognitive impairment was correlated with pattern shift VEP (PSVEP) alterations [76]. Of 33 head-injured patients tested with PSVEP: 50% of patients with severe cognitive dysfunction had abnormal PSVEP compared with only 11% with mild cognitive impairment and 39% with moderate cognitive impairment. Moreover, the mean of both P_{100} latency and interocular P_{100} latency difference was significantly abnormal in the head trauma group compared to the control group [76]. According to another study, patients with symptomatic post-concussion syndrome had mildly abnormal flash-VEP which was seen more clearly at higher stimulation frequencies [164].

However, asymptomatic concussed patients had nearly normal VEP which was mainly of low amplitude with asymmetry. The ability to follow the VEP at a higher frequency was correlated with clinical recovery [164].

LESION LOCALIZATION

Physiological localization of a lesion may be undertaken by using appropriate EP modalities and knowledge of the anatomical generator source of each peak (Tables 6.2 and 6.3). As mentioned above, an abnormal BAEP and SSEP in head-injured patients generally indicates brainstem dysfunction, whereas a longer latency SEP, VEP, and AEP may indicate cerebral or cortical dysfunction [34,72,156] (Table 6.4).

Associated BAEP changes with various brainstem lesions of the ascending auditory pathway was studied extensively in the cat. Section of auditory nerve at the internal acoustic meatus produced ipsilateral absence of BAEP beyond wave I. Destruction of the cochlear nucleus caused ipsilateral loss of wave II and subsequent waves, whereas damage beyond the cochlear nucleus caused ipsilateral loss of all waves beyond wave II. Extensive lesions to the superior olivary complex – including the decussating fibers of the trapezoid body – resulted in ipsilateral loss of wave III and subsequent waves with attenuation of the contralateral response. Lesions beyond the superior olivary complex showed preservation of wave III and loss of subsequent peaks. Injury to the inferior colliculus caused marked changes to wave V, but not the earlier waves while damage rostral to the inferior colliculus did not produce significant alteration of wave V [1,28,102].

BAEP

BAEP findings have been reported in human pathological lesions and intraoperative brainstem recording in humans [90,91,158,198,199,209]. BAEP can provide reliable information concerning the site of the lesion as well as the degree of involvement of auditory pathways (Table 6.2). Wave I, III, and V BAEP peaks are stable and often useful indicators of auditory pathway integrity [37]. Prolongation of both peak V latency and I-V IPL was often found in patients with various brainstem pathologic conditions [42,196,203,209]. On the other hand, all five peaks were intact in patients with cerebral or cerebellar lesions [191,192,198].

In over 100 patients studied, abnormalities of each BAEP component were correlated with postmortem and radiologic localization of brainstem lesions [201]. Alteration or loss of wave I was correlated with an auditory nerve lesion, wave II with pontomedullary lesions, wave III with caudal pontine lesions, wave IV with rostral pontine or midbrain lesions, wave V with midbrain lesions, wave VI with thalamic lesions, and wave VII with thalamic or thalamocortical lesions [158,196,198,199,201,209,213]. Abnormal BAEP was found in all patients with pontine lesions [91]. Significant delay of the mean latencies of wave III and V was observed and in particular a prolonged latency of wave V was seen in midbrain lesions [91].

Preservation of waves I and III with absence of wave V bilaterally was reported in two patients with rostral pontine tegmental hematomas [27]. Lesions in the ventral pons that spare the auditory tracts in the dorsal pontine tegmentum (as in patients with "locked-in" syndrome) were associated with intact BAEP [27,160]. The same investigators reported a normal BAEP recording in patients with lateral medullary syndrome. Traumatic midbrain injury was associated with altered BAEP wave V, even before the lesion was visualized on CT scan [179].

BAEP testing was done in two patients with unilateral gunshot wounds to the pons. In one case, BAEP was reported as normal, which indicated sparing of the adjacent superior olivary complex and lateral lemniscus [40]. In the second case, ipsilateral BAEP showed loss of waves II and III, suggesting damage of the superior olivary complex [23]. These investigators concluded that the clinical findings, neuroradiographic features, operative course, and evoked response data correlated with the functional anatomy of the pons.

Asymmetries of bilaterally recorded BAEPs may refer to a unilateral brainstem lesion or a lesion affecting the crossed auditory projection. Nevertheless, abnormality of BAEP is usually ipsilateral to the brainstem lesion [91,160]. However an abnormal BAEP recorded contralateral to the side of lesion was noted in some reports [27,144].

BAEP was reported to provide more reliable early information regarding brainstem function than neurological signs or CT scan findings [91,179,198,199,202,212]. Primary brainstem injury and hidden lesions can be diagnosed by BAEPs [212]. Intrinsic traumatic brainstem lesions may be associated with increased latency of waves III-V and suppression of waves II-V, whereas extrinsic brainstem compression produced an increase in all latencies and interpeak latencies [91]. In one study, there was a poor correlation between BAEP findings and brainstem lesions as revealed by the CT scan [112]. Yet, many clinicians feel that serial BAEP recordings are useful to follow patients with brainstem lesions.

SEP

In animal studies, SEPs showed a decrease in amplitude over the side of a subdural hematoma [164]. In the experimentally rotated monkey, pre-impact SEPs disappeared at the time of impact and throughout the comatose period. Recovery of the second peak (P_2) occurred with arousal of the animal from coma. There was a marked increase in percent delay of P_2 conduction in rotated animals compared to the unimpaired linear translated group. In the latter, P_2 was always present [164].

SEP recording can be helpful in the clinical diagnosis of peripheral nerve, brachial plexus, spinal cord, brainstem, thalamic and cortical lesions [13,67,104,159]. Avulsion injury of dorsal spinal roots was associated with intact P_9 and absence of subsequent SEP peaks [14]. Hemisection at the level of bulbo-spinal junction produced loss of

SEP components beyond N/P$_{13}$ [136]. P$_{14}$ and N$_{18}$ waves may still be seen in patients with thalamic, radiation, or cortical lesions [14]. Alteration of N$_{14}$ or N$_{18}$ has been seen in patients with a brainstem lesion [14,90] and it was suggested that N$_{18}$ of SEP could be used for brainstem monitoring [14,46]. In one study, the absence of N$_{19}$ and a prolonged P/N$_{13}$-N$_{19}$ was noted in 8 of 15 patients with pontine or midbrain lesions [13]. The absence of SEP waves beyond P/N$_{13}$ was seen in patients with pontine, midbrain, or total brain death [34].

Asymmetry of the SEP was seen in patients with unilateral lesions affecting the sensory pathway [34,64,119,120]. Focal destructive hemispheric lesions may affect SEPs recorded over the affected lobe or side [64,118,124,217]. SEPs were also found to be abnormal in patients with thalamic insults (hemorrhage, infarction), particularly when CT scan failed to demonstrate the lesion [116,137]. Ipsilateral delay in SEP latency and waveform changes (monophasic) were also reported in patients with compressive intracranial hematomas [119]. SEP abnormalities were correlated with the severity of these lesions [64,217]. A study was done correlating type of intracranial lesion and SEP findings. Compressive lesions, i.e., subdural hematomas, were associated with loss of waveform complexity and delayed latency. Ischemia was associated with amplitude suppression; hematomas, with changes in waveform morphology [17,119,120]. These distinctions are not usually possible.

Abnormal sensory EPs recorded in the post-injury period may relate to a reversible functional disturbance and not necessarily an overt structural abnormality. Persistent EP abnormalities may point to irreversible peripheral or central nervous system damage [129,183]. Brain or spinal cord edema may also contribute to EP abnormalities after injury. It should be remembered, however, that lesions sparing auditory or somatosensory (dorsal column, lemniscal) pathways may be associated with normal BAEP or SEP, respectively [13,27,160].

VEP AND MEP

Visual pathway abnormalities can be detected by VEPs. Anterior visual pathway dysfunction and possibly posterior visual impairment can be diagnosed early using pattern reversal VEPs [87]. Abnormalities of early VEP components may indicate lesions involving the primary visual system [143]. However, in our experience, orbital swelling from frontal or temporal impacts may not allow adequate visual stimulation in these acute injuries.

Multimodality EPs were reported to be useful in localizing lesions [71,188]. A positive correlation between the location of neuroanatomical lesions at autopsy or operation and the location of traumatic brain dysfunction detected by MEPs was found. Occipital lesions were found to correlate well with VEP findings, parietal lobe lesions with SEP, temporal lobe lesions with VEP and AEP, diencephalic lesions with SEP, and brainstem lesions with SSEP and BAEP. On the other hand, frontal lobe lesions failed to show correlation with MEPs [71]. With an abnormal BAEP or SSEP, later waves (AEP, SEP) may be absent or abnormal.

INTRACRANIAL PRESSURE AND HERNIATION

Several studies in animals and humans have shown that measurements of BAEP waves I, III, IV, and V, and the III-V and I-V IPLs, may be sensitive indicators of increased intracranial pressure and transtentorial herniation (Tables 6.5and 6.6). Generally very high ICP or actual brainstem shift has been required to consistently produce these abnormalities.

Animal Studies: BAEP, SEP, SSEP

Elevations of CSF pressure by spinal catheter infusion of isotonic saline in cats has been associated with measurable changes in the electrical potentials generated from the cochlea (ECochG). These changes were associated with elevations in perilymphatic pressure transmitted from the CSF [7,8,58,110]. The increase in perilymphatic pressure was associated with parallel distortions and threshold shift in the ECochG [7,29,58,122,138]. It remains possible that cochlear abnormalities secondary to increased CSF pressure could be reflected in wave I and later BAEP waves.

Animal studies have been helpful regarding BAEP abnormalities accompanying brain herniation. Measurement of wave V was useful in predicting transtentorial herniation and early brainstem dysfunction in cats and monkeys with supratentorial balloon inflation [145,205]. Waves IV and V were progressively suppressed by increasing the balloon volume while earlier BAEP components were less affected. Gradual recovery of BAEPs in the reverse order occurred after deflation of the balloon. A marked depression of wave V (30% of control) followed by complete absence of wave V was correlated with the beginning and completion of transtentorial herniation, respectively [146]. During acute expansion of a balloon in the posterior fossa of cats, changes in amplitude of waves III and V were useful in detecting upward transtentorial herniation of the midbrain and foraminal herniation of cerebellum [147]. Wave III was considered a sensitive index for predicting medullary failure in that setting. In the cat and monkey model, recovery of BAEP changes was also reported upon lowering ICP by balloon deflation [145,205].

Gradual inflation of a supratentorial balloon in cats showed that late components of SEPs were suppressed first, followed by the early components of the SEPs, then wave V and IV of the BAEP in that order. However, SEPs did not recover as did BAEP upon release of pressure. The investigators concluded that the late SEP components were found to be the earliest and most severely affected potentials during transtentorial herniation followed by BAEPS [145]. Similar findings were reported in monkeys [205].

Table 6.5. Evoked Potential Findings Suggestive of Brainstem and Hemispheric Dysfunction

| | Dysfunction | |
	Brainstem	Hemispheric
BAEP	Abnormal	Normal
SSEP	Abnormal	Normal
LLAEP, MLAEP	Normal	Abnormal
MLSEP, LLSEP	Normal	Abnormal
VEP	Normal	Abnormal

BAEP: Brainstem Auditory Evoked Potential; SSEP: Short Latency Somatosensory Evoked Potential; MLAEP and LLAEP: Middle and Long Latency Auditory Evoked Potential; MLSEP and LLSEP: Middle and Long Latency Somatosensory Evoked Potential; VEP: Visual Evoked Potential.

Table 6.6. Reported Changes in Auditory Evoked Potentials Associated with Elevated Intracranial Pressure and Early Herniation

Depressed cortical AEP
Depression and latency delay waves IV or V
Latency delay wave III
Prolonged interpeak latencies I-V, III-V
Latency delay wave I

Initial increase in the amplitude of different BAEP peaks as well as delay in latencies and IPLs was recorded in cats with induced intracranial hypertension [113,114]. Progressive elevation of ICP by supratentorial balloon inflation was associated with increased IPLs and latency of single BAEP components in a rostrocaudal fashion. Wave V was lost first and did not recover with release of pressure, then wave III was lost but recovered with release of pressure. At the stage of respiratory paralysis, cochlear response was still recorded and release of pressure did not cause reappearance of the remaining BAEP [113,114].

Marked reduction of inferior collicular blood flow was experimentally observed during uncal herniation in the cat [151] and monkey [unpublished data]. During induced uncal herniation by gradual inflation of a supratentorial balloon in these animals, a marked reduction of blood flow was observed in the thalamus, inferior colliculus, and medulla oblongata — in that order.

Marked elevation of ICP in cats and rabbits resulted in latency and amplitude changes in the BAEP [135,140,176]. The waveforms were abolished when the levels of ICP exceeded CBF, and became irreversible unless the CBF was corrected [176]. Prolongation of I-III IPL was also reported to correlate with the ICP level in rabbits with increased ICP by CSF infusion [140]. In another study, hydrocephalic rabbits underwent BAEP testing [61]. The baseline BAEP of a normal rabbit included positive peaks P_0-P_1 to P_5 and negative peaks N_1 to N_5 were studied. BAEP changes observed when average ICP was 38 mmH$_2$O (normal 25 mmH$_2$O) included increased peaks N_2, P_2, and P_5 latencies, P_1-P_5 IPL, and increased wave I and decreased V amplitudes. When ICP was further elevated acutely by CSF infusion (250, 500, 700 mmH2O), significant delay of peaks P_0, P_1, N_2, P_3, N_4, and N_5, prolonged P_1-P_3, P_3-P_5, and P_1-P_5 IPLs, and decrease of wave IV amplitude were seen. It was concluded that changes in absolute latencies of P_0-N_2 as well as absolute latencies of subsequent waves were possibly explained by cochlear changes secondary to high ICP, whereas changes in IPLs were best explained by a neuropraxic pressure effect on the brainstem [61].

Several experimental studies in the cat showed no correlation between BAEP changes and elevated ICP [135,206]. Others believed cerebral perfusion pressure rather than ICP determined BAEP changes [68]. In a cat study yielding elevated ICP by mock CSF infusion, maintenance of adequate CPP resulted in no change in BAEPs [68]. An abnormal BAEP was recorded only when CPP was below a critically low value and recovery of BAEP following elevation of CPP was also noted [68]. It was found that at CPP values which suppressed the EEG and late somatosensory evoked potentials, BAEP did not show any significant changes. However, at very low CPP, BAEP components beyond wave I were lost [193,194]. BAEP was resistant not only to high ICP, but also to marked hypoxia and hypoglycemia [49]. Furthermore, BAEP and SSEP recordings in cats did not show any change in the setting of either ventricular dilation or increased ICP [206]. Only preterminally when there was marked compromise of CPP due to high ICP were EP changes seen [206].

It was reported that in cats, induced high ICP by either epidural balloon inflation or intraventricular infusion produced more marked depression in higher centers of the auditory pathway than in lower ones [135]. Cortical AEPs were affected early by high ICP. The recovery of AEP was much slower than that of the early components after release of intracranial pressure. The conclusion of this study was that cortical and subcortical potentials were most sensitive to high ICP followed by potentials recorded from the medial geniculate body, inferior colliculus, and cochlear nucleus (most resistant). Recovery was noted in the reverse order after release of intracranial pressure [135]. Significant changes in cortical and subcortical auditory responses were also confirmed in a study of increased ICP in the rabbit [140]. A study in rats showed the reliability of SEP changes with increasing ICP [218].

Animal Studies: VEP

Some laboratory studies have suggested that increased ICP and ventricular enlargement may be reflected by the VEP [39,74,177,215]. A study was carried out in dogs with induced intracranial hypertension by infusion of mock cerebral spinal fluid into the ventricle [39]. Changes in visual evoked potentials correlated well with CPP and lateral sinus venous O_2 saturation secondary to elevated ICP [39]. In a study using baboons, a significant correlation was found between the amplitude of the direct parieto-occipital cortical response (DCR), and both CPP and CBF rather than high ICP per se [74]. The ICP was elevated by mock CSF infusion through the cisterne magna. A closer correlation between CBF and DCR amplitude than between CPP and DCR was seen. DCR was abolished when CBF was lower than 40% of the control. SEP did not show significant changes. It was concluded that the effect of high ICP on DCR was primarily mediated through CBF [74].

BAEP, AEP, SSEP in Humans

Several studies have been carried out in humans and the results have agreed to an extent with the above mentioned animal model findings. In recent BAEP studies on patients with supratentorial mass lesions, wave V absolute latency prolongation was noted before pupillary changes [4,144,152]. Auditory sensitivity, measured in patients with raised intracranial tension, is known to deteriorate by about 30 dB and return to normal following surgical decompression in a few small studies [18,184]. This deterioration in hearing may reflect changes in perilymphatic pressures in response to raised ICP [31]. BAEP changes were marked when ICP approached 30 mmHg. Following the lowering of ICP with 200 ml of 10% glycerol given intravenously, shortening or normalization of a prolonged wave V absolute latency was demonstrated in almost all patients with anisocoria with or without clinical improvement of uncal herniation. Inconsistent III-V IPL prolongation was also noted [144].

Wave V absolute latency prolongation as a result of high ICP and early signs of uncal herniation was also reported in another series of 12 patients [148]. Efforts to lower ICP by 10% glycerol administration were successful in normalizing wave V latency with or without clinical improvement. Suppression of wave V and prolongation of I-V IPL were noted earlier than clinical deterioration in three patients with brain stem compression secondary to supratentorial lesions. Administration of steroids caused normalization of wave V latency in two of the three tumor patients. Wave V changes were found to correlate with rostrocaudal deterioration of brainstem function and wave V recovery was delayed compared to the earlier BAEP components [108,148,149,152]. Generally ICP elevations above 35 to 40 mmHg for 24 hours were necessary for BAEP changes such as I-V IPL prolongation [108].

BAEP abnormalities can be helpful in the detection of transtentorial herniation at different stages of progression. The upper brainstem was reported to be more vulnerable than the lower brainstem during clinical rostrocaudal deterioration [101]. The presence of brainstem rotation or foreshortening on CT scan was found to correlate with prolongation of the I-V IPL (> 4.48 msec) [57]. Compression of the cisterns around the brainstem noted by CT scan may cause delay in III-V IPL. However, 45% of 59 patients with normal BAEP had basal cistern compression, as noted by CT scan [130]. In another study, the CT scan of patients with normal BAEP or prolonged I-V IPL (not greater than 4.48 msec) showed only basal cistern obliteration with or without contralateral temporal horn dilatation. On the other hand, the CT scan of patients with prolonged I-V IPL (> 4.48 msec) or absence of all components beyond wave I showed more severe brainstem deformation [224].

BAEP changes, including prolongation of III-V and I-V IPL, suppression of wave V, and absence of wave VI and VII were reported in 8 of 20 patients with supratentorial tumors and clinical signs of increased ICP [20]. In a patient with a large supratentorial meningioma, BAEP wave latency was reported to be an early sign associated with high ICP [190]. Elevated BAEP threshold was also noted in 70% of hydrocephalic patients; it improved later in some of the patients as soon as the ICP was corrected [115]. The most common abnormal response in these latter patients was distortion of wave V. Wave V was broadened and lacked its characteristic following reverse slope [115]. In a similar study of 16 hydrocephalic babies, both waves I and V showed prolonged latency and depressed amplitude [52]. V/I ratio was significantly reduced. Elevated BAEP threshold was also noted. However, I-V IPL did not show marked changes. Of all BAEP abnormalities, reduction of wave V amplitude presented the most common abnormality. Improvement of BAEP was noted in some patients on the follow-up testing [52]. Furthermore, depression of wave V amplitude and prolongation of I-V IPL were observed in a hydrocephalic neonate, which improved after shunting [48].

Forty-one patients with impending transtentorial herniation underwent binaural BAEP recorded between Cz and the mastoid ipsilateral to a lateralized lesion [152]. Non-survivors showed prolongation of wave V absolute latency and I-V IPL. Prolongation of wave I latency was found to be a consistent finding in those who died compared to those who survived. In the early third nerve states of transtentorial herniation, I-III and I-V IPLs were within normal limits. In the midbrain-upper pons stage, I-V IPL was increased and no patients survived. Finally, in the medullary stage, waves III and V were absent and also no patients survived. There was good general correlation between ICP and BAEP latencies over the course of transtentorial herniation. BAEP peaks disappeared as the ICP reached its highest level and the reduction of ICP was associated with shortening of IPLs. Therefore, absolute BAEP latencies and IPLs were thought to be sensitive indicators in early detection of brain stem dysfunction [152].

As in several animal studies [39,49,68,74,135,193,194,206], some investigators concluded that there was no relation between BAEP changes and ICP in humans [107,109]. However, others have found that CPP was the crucial factor rather than ICP alone [68,84,108]. Very high ICP values (64 mmHg) did not affect BAEP recorded from children as long as the CPP was maintained above 30 mmHg. Recovery of BAEP abnormalities occurred as soon as the CPP was corrected [68]. Low CPP is believed to produce brainstem ischemia which results in BAEP abnormalities. Moreover, BAEP was found to be more resistent than EEG and SSEP to low CPP. Mildly low CPP values suppressed EEG and the late components of SEPs, but significant changes were not yet observed in BAEP. Only at very low CPP did BAEP show significant changes [193,194].

It has been our experience that elevations of ICP in the clinical range frequently encountered, in the absence of brainstem shift, do not significantly alter routine

BAEP in patients with intracranial lesions. Yet laboratory and some clinical evidence exists that cochlear function is affected by elevated ICP.

Extensive study of latency and amplitude versus stimulus intensity functions of wave V may reflect cochlear abnormalities. Accordingly, the authors developed a modified BAEP (MBAEP) technique in an attempt to enhance the sensitivity of BAEP in patients with intracranial mass lesions and clinical signs of mild to moderately elevated ICP [63,204]. Our MBAEP method is a binaural, rapid rate (70.4/sec) BAEP performed at four different levels of moderate intensity (65, 72, 75, 85 dBpeSPL). This method was followed in 106 symptomatic patients with clinical and radiologic or invasively recorded mild to moderately increased ICP and was compared with the Standard BAEP at 75 and 110 dBSPL. The patients were divided according to the etiology of increased ICP into trauma (53%) and non-trauma (47%) groups. Normal values were obtained from 35 matched controls. MBAEP (including latency/intensity and amplitude/intensity measures) was abnormal in 93 of 106 patients (88%) whereas standard BAEP at 75 dB and 110 dB (including wave V latency and amplitude measures) was abnormal in almost half of the patients. Furthermore, the normal linear or curvilinear relationship between wave V latency or amplitude and stimulus intensity was disturbed in the patient population. Instead, a translocated or an irregular shaped curve was seen representing a disturbed wave V latency or amplitude/intensity function. Normal BAEP was recorded in 30% to 40% of patients in whom MBAEP was abnormal. No case was found with an abnormal BAEP but normal MBAEP. Common MBAEP abnormalities in these patients included wave V latency/intensity dysfunction (75%, amplitude depression (62%), and absolute latency prolongation (42%). Therefore the latency/intensity abnormality was thought to be a suggestive indicator of elevated ICP. Also, wave V absolute latency and amplitude of MBAEP and BAEP showed a statistical difference among the normal, trauma, and non-trauma groups. Another remarkable finding was the loss of waves I and/or III peaks (25% to 50%) in pathologic cases compared to normal controls. There was good agreement between normalization of MBAEP-BAEP and ICP correction [63].

Only a few studies in humans are available correlating high ICP and SEP or AEP. AEPs (middle and long latency auditory potentials) were abnormal in 6 of 15 hydrocephalic patients [50]. P_{300} of AEP was significantly altered in a patient with marked hydrocephalus due to congenital aqueductal stenosis despite nearly normal VEP, BAEP, and middle latency auditory responses (MLR) [219]. SEP recording was normal in hydrocephalic patients despite abnormal VEP [139].

VEP in Humans

Several studies in patients with hydrocephalus and increased ICP had shown definite VEP alterations which tend to normalize later after CSF diversion [6,50,54, 59,77,78,99,139,141,165,189,222,223].

In patients with hydrocephalus or brain edema, a linear relationship was found between ICP levels (> 300 mmH$_2$O; 39 mmHg) and a latency shift of the N$_2$ wave of flash evoked visual potentials [222,223]. VEP changes included delay latency of P$_{100}$, abnormal waveform, asymmetries, and fatiguability to increasing stimulus frequency [189]. Reduction of P$_{100}$ latency was seen post-shunting, however worsening of VEP was associated with progression of hydrocephalus [189]. Pattern-shift (reversal) VEP was an excellent indicator for visual pathway dysfunction in patients with hydrocephalus [6]. In 10 patients with hydrocephalus, 6 had abnormal VEP configuration and 2 had delayed latency [139]. Following ventriculo-peritoneal shunting, normalization of VEP was only seen in those with abnormal VEP configuration [139]. Delayed latency of P$_{100}$ was thought to be seen frequently in infants developing hydrocephalus before 56 weeks of age [77]. Significant prolongation of P$_{100}$ was also observed in infants with enlarged heads and brain damage. Recovery of P$_{100}$ after shunting was seen mostly in patients with normal mental status regardless of ventricular size. Therefore, the investigators suggested that serial VEP recording would be helpful in assessing the mental development in this particular setting [77]. The same investigators noted that VEP alteration was consistently seen in infants with both ventriculomegaly and enlargement of the head and in addition a slow return of P$_{100}$ to normal values after shunting [78]. Flash-VEP was abnormal in 8 of 15 hydrocephalic patients, whereas AEP was abnormal in 6 patients and 4 had both abnormal VEP and AEP [50].

Other studies showed VEP changes in patients with papilledema and benign intracranial hypertension [96,111]. On the other hand, some believed that a poor correlation exists between papilledema, benign intracranial hypertension, and VEP [15,16,34,86,88,182]. Further confirmation of relative VEP changes due to increased ICP is needed and this may well prove a fruitful line of investigation.

EVOKED POTENTIALS AS A PROGNOSTIC SIGN

Serial clinical examination provides the most accurate prediction of outcome in severely head-injured patients. However, sensory EPs may enhance the accuracy of outcome prediction, particularly when clinical findings are unclear. Moreover, evoked potential – BAEP in particular – was found a reliable measure in those patients who are in barbiturate coma or therapeutically paralyzed, or when the clinical examination is not obtainable [84,126,130,131]. Evoked potential results were believed by many authors to be more reliable than clinical findings and no false pessimistic predictions were encountered [12,107,154].

Sensory EPs may give an accurate prediction of the patient's outcome in the early post-injury period [105,166,187]. Mechanical brain trauma and edema may cause EP changes recorded in the early post-injury period [129]. These EP abnormalities may recover at a later time emphasizing the importance of serial and delayed EP recording in predicting outcome.

Table 6.7. Evoked Potential Modalities Recommended in Literature for Predicting Outcome

BAEP alone
BAEP and AEP
SSEP alone
SSEP and BAEP
SEP and BAEP
SEP and VEP
MEP

BAEP: Brainstem Auditory Evoked Potential; AEP: Auditory Evoked Potential; SSEP: Short Latency Somatosensory Evoked Potential; SEP: Somatosensory Evoked Potential; VEP: Visual Evoked Potential; MEP: Multimodality Evoked Potential.

Table 6.8. Evoked Potential Findings Associated with Unfavorable Outcome

Consistant abnormality(ies)
Gross (multiple) abnormalities
Abnormality(ies) detected in more than one modality
Absence of peak(s)
Prolonged interpeak latencies
Prolonged central conduction time
Reversed amplitude ratio

Repeated grossly abnormal sensory evoked potentials usually indicate an unfavorable outcome, and consistently normal potentials often predict favorable outcome. Mildly abnormal EP may not be as helpful in prognostication. Serial monitoring is required for accurate prediction of outcome and further EP changes may relate to deterioration or improvement in the patient's condition. Reversible abnormalities as a result of aggressive management may or may not indicate improvement in the ultimate outcome [84] (Tables 6.7 and 6.8).

BAEP

Although the type of sensory EPs used to evaluate head injury prognosis has varied (Table 6.7), many investigators believe that BAEP is a useful prognostic indicator in head-injured patients [12,51,57,81,83,142,168,185,187,211,212]. These investigators and others recommend the use of a combination of BAEPs and AEP (middle and long latency auditory potentials) as predictors of outcome [82,83,84,105,106,107, 166,180].

BAEP is a sensitive indicator of the functional integrity of the brainstem [25,191, 212]. Absence of all BAEP components or absence of all components beyond wave I or II usually indicates poor outcome and is often irreversible [25,51,82,83,84, 113,129,142,166,180,185,191,212,220].

Gross BAEP abnormalities were frequently seen in traumatized patients with an unfavorable outcome [81,83,106,107,168]. Absence of wave IV, V, or all BAEP peaks carried a worse prognosis than simply a delay in latencies [134]. Marked exaggeration of wave I amplitude compared to other waves was seen in cases with severe brainstem dysfunction [80,84,142,199]. In another study, all patients with absent IV-V or earlier waves died [51]. Moreover, prognosis was worse in patients with both delayed wave V and I-V interpeak latencies and reduced V/I amplitude ratio [51].

However, normal to mildly abnormal BAEP was often associated with favorable outcome [82,106,107,142,166]. Absence or delayed latency of wave V may be observed in patients with a favorable outcome and may often be reversible. Absence of wave V with subsequent step-wise loss of V, IV, and III peaks at less than 12 hours following injury was associated with an unfavorable outcome [129,194,211,212].

Timing of BAEP testing as well as repeated recordings were helpful in reflecting the severity and progression of brainstem injury and in predicting outcome [212]. Patients with prolonged I-V IPLs were graded better than patients with absence of wave V [142,166]. Patients with a high IV-V/I amplitude ratio were more likely to have a favorable outcome [185]. I-V IPL was found to be a sensitive predictor of outcome in severe head-injured patients [57]. Favorable outcome was noted in patients with I-V IPL < 4.48 msec compared with an unfavorable outcome in those with I-V IPL > 4.48 msec (normal I-V IPL 4.03 + 0.17) [57]. In 30 head trauma patients there was a correlation between III-V IPL and poor outcome. Prolonged I-III IPL was associated with grave prognosis [185].

Consistent gross BAEP abnormalities, especially wave V latency, may indicate severe diffuse axonal injury (DAI) associated with poor outcome. On the other hand, normalization of BAEP abnormalities was seen in those patients who survived [62].

An abnormal BAEP recording was a better predictor of unfavorable outcome than a normal test for predicting a favorable outcome [12,30,84,105,130,168]. However, it has been reported that patients with bilateral normal BAEP responses had the best chance of survival [51]. In one study, it was estimated that overall predictive accuracy of BAEP was 50% [81]. By contrast, another BAEP study in post-traumatic patients showed an overall predictive accuracy of 77%, or 91% if deaths from extracranial causes were excluded [25].

Spectral energy analysis of recorded auditory frequency bands is a recently introduced method which may expand our understanding of auditory evoked potentials [79]. In spectral analysis, BAEP amplitude is described in the frequency domain. A recent investigation analyzed the spectral content of BAEP in 70 comatose patients. This group, especially those with head injury, demonstrated less overall BAEP spectral power (voltage) compared to a normal group. The spectral content of BAEP varied according to patient outcome [79].

BAEP, MLR, AEP

Patients with preservation of middle and long latency potentials (AEP) had a favorable outcome [105,106,180]. These later auditory potentials could be significant measures of communicative/cognitive outcome in head trauma patients. Favorable outcome was also observed in patients with intact long, middle, and short latency potentials compared to those with only short latency (BAEP) responses [105,106, 180]. Normalization of BAEPs have been correlated with recovery from the post-concussion syndrome [19].

The P300 (msec) (auditory) evoked potential was strongly correlated with neuro-psychological evaluation, useful to confirm cognitive impairment and residual brain dysfunction. The P300 was also found to correlate with post-traumatic amnesia [167].

BAEP and middle latency responses (MLR, 10 to 50 msec) may enhance accuracy of prognosis [80,82,84,105,106,130,166,180]. Consistently normal MLR within 10 days post injury was reported to indicate good neurological and communicative outcome, whereas consistently abnormal MLR indicated poor outcome even with a normal BAEP [84,166]. However, as mentioned above, MLR can be altered by medications and other factors. The outcome of patients with an increased BAEP I-V IPL was found to be related to MLR results and to subsequent improvement of auditory waveforms within the first three months after injury [166].

Fifty-four comatose patients were assessed with short, middle, and long latency AEPs within 72 hours after admission [105]. Survival rate was 100% in patients with normal potentials, 91% in patients with only an absence of long latency potentials, 60% in patients with only intact short latency potentials (BAEP), 10% in patients with abnormal BAEP and absent subsequent potentials, and no survival of patients with absence of all auditory potentials. Every patient with altered or obliterated BAEP had absent subsequent potentials. These investigators deduced that a normal middle latency potential was clearly a predictor of survival in comatose patients, whereas a normal BAEP was not a reliable predictor of survival. Abnormal or absent BAEP was a reliable predictor of death [105]. The addition of clinical findings to BAEP and AEP (neurophysiological scale) was found to predict the outcome more accurately and with no false pessimistic predictions [107].

SEPs

Somatosensory evoked potentials are thought to be a reliable predictor of favorable or unfavorable outcome from head injury [12,30,45,98,130,131,171,173,183,216]. It has recently been reported that SSEPS were more vulnerable to central nervous system trauma than BAEPs and VEPs [12,30, 126]. In addition, normal BAEPs have been reported in patients with severely abnormal SSEPs [30].

Trauma patients with eight identifiable SEP wave peaks in the first 300 msec had a better outcome than those with only five peaks, whereas no recovery was reported in patients with only two primary SEP peaks [45]. Absence of early components had a worse prognostic value than absence of later components only (provided no barbiturates or sedatives were given). The majority of patients with absence of all components or absence of all components beyond P_{15} died [45,73,129,171,183,216].

SEPs have been correlated with outcome in 75% to 80% of head trauma patients. Improvement of SEP was seen in patients with good recovery, whereas consistently abnormal SEPs were recorded in disabled patients [98].

Central conduction time (CCT = N_{20} − N_{14}) of SEP has been correlated with patients' outcome after head injury [30,98,126,128,173,183,216]. In addition, CCT was found to be more resistant to barbiturates than later SEP components [129,134]. In a recent study of 101 patients with severe head injury, CCT was not much better than the neurological examination regarding outcome prediction [126]. However CCT provided prognostic information in paralyzed or sedated patients [126].

Normal CCT and amplitude ratio between the peak of N_{20} and the subsequent positivity and the peak of N_{14} and its subsequent positivity were found in trauma patients with good outcome [183]. Prolonged CCT and decreased amplitude ratio were correlated with poor outcome. The most prolonged CCT was seen in patients who died. Asymmetries of SEPs were seen in patients with moderate to severe disability [183]. Early normalization of CCT and amplitude ratio was found in patients with favorable outcome. Patients with primary brainstem injury who had a good recovery might demonstrate asymmetric or absent SEPs and increased CCT [173,183].

In another study, bilateral absence of the N_{20}-P_{23} complex was associated with poor outcome and the majority of these patients met the clinical criteria of brain death [133,134]. The length of survival was correlated partly with the presence or absence of BAEP and brainstem reflexes. Patients with only BAEP wave I or no response, survived 8 to 46 days. Patients with unilateral delay in N_{14}-N_{20} conduction had a favorable outcome compared to patients with bilateral N_{14}-N_{20} delay [133,134].

Patients with unilateral or bilateral absence of N_{20} within the first four days had an unfavorable outcome [30]. Preservation of N_{20}/P_{23} implied a good prognosis, whereas loss of N_{20}/P_{23} implied poor prognosis [69].

Long latency SEPs were correlated with the patient's clinical status and outcome [169]. Normal long latency SEPs indicated favorable outcome, whereas missing or questionable long latency SEPs was an unfavorable sign (provided no barbiturates of sedatives were given). A return of consciousness and improvement of neurological status correlated with return of the late SEP components [169]. In another report, the appearance of long latency SEPs during emergence from coma was compatible with a more optimistic outcome [171].

VEPs

A study of visual evoked potentials in head trauma patients showed that flash-VEP was a good indicator of unfavorable outcome, but false pessimistic predictions were present [12]. A study of monocular pattern-reversal VEPs was found to correlate with cognitive function in awake post-traumatic patients. P100 latency prolongation was the most common finding [76].

Abnormalities were more clearly seen at the higher VEP stimulation frequencies [163,164]. Recovery was frequently underway when VEP was able to follow a faster rate of stimulation. Retro-retinal conduction dysfunction tends to cause latency prolongation and visual acuity impairment may produce amplitude depression.

In another study of brain damaged patients, long latency VEPs were reported to correlate with psychosocial disability [175]. Mildly abnormal VEPs were found in patients with post-traumatic syndrome [76,163,164,175]. But severe hemispheric dysfunction was usually present if VEPs were preserved in the occipital region only. A gradual spreading of VEP over the scalp tended to indicate improvement in brain function [171].

Multimodality Evoked Potentials

Severely head-injured patients have been studied with multiple EP modalities (MEP). In one study, auditory, somatosensory, and visual cortical evoked potentials were well correlated with outcome, whereas short latency brainstem potentials alone did not correlate with outcome [125]. The above investigators found that simply counting the number of identifiable waves present was the optimal method for analyzing the data. The fewer the number of wave peaks, the poorer the outcome [125]. Later cortical components of each modality correlated with the level of consciousness and depth of coma [71].

A combination of SEPs and BAEPs was a more reliable indicator of outcome than either EP alone [129]. Short latency SEP was found to be a powerful prognostic indicator in the early post-injury period whereas BAEP was significantly correlated to later outcome [71]. A combination of SEP-BAEP [30,126,129] or SEP-VEP [171] has also been suggested. MEPs with a specific grading scale for auditory, somatosensory, visual evoked potentials was thought to give the most accurate results [70,188]. MEP recording appears to be an excellent prognostic indicator as the functional integrity of three different sensory pathways is assessed [71,125].

Graded MEPs predicted outcome in 100 severely head-injured patients with approximately 100% accuracy, excluding patients who died from systemic causes (80% without exclusion) [73]. Mildly abnormal MEPs were predictive of good to moderate outcome in 81% of the patients, whereas severe to absent MEPs indicated a poor outcome in 76% of patients. A linear relationship was found between severity of MEP abnormality and a less favorable outcome. Severely abnormal MEPs (the last grade in the scale) was maximally predictive of poor outcome regardless of any other factors [73].

In patients with acute subdural hematoma, MEP was a clear indicator not only for outcome prediction but also for early detection of reversible and irreversible brainstem dysfunction [188].

In 133 severely head-injured patients, MEPs were the most reliable predictor for outcome [154]. The accuracy rate was 91% and there were no false pessimistic predictions. When clinical and MEP data were combined together, the accuracy rate became 89% with 4% false pessimistic predictions. By contrast, clinical data alone predicted outcome with 82% accuracy and 9% false pessimistic predictions [154].

A follow-up one year post-injury study was carried out using MEPs [157]. Patients with consistently normal MEPs had good recovery, whereas patients with consistently absent potentials had poor outcome. Patients with stable or improving mildly abnormal MEPs had favorable outcome despite complications. Patients with severe MEP abnormalities which later improved had a favorable outcome, while those with persistent or deteriorating severe EP abnormalities had poor outcome. The changes found in serial MEPs were better prognostic indicators than the presence or absence of complications. MEP changes (deterioration or improvement) may at times precede changes in the patient's clinical status [157].

EP monitoring may be useful in confirming brain death [13,69,80,113,196]. Before interpreting EP findings in brain death, peripheral sensory system integrity must be assessed. This testing can be done through recording wave I or II of the BAEP, and Erbs potential and P/N_{15} of the SSEP [69,70,71]. Preservation of P/N_{13} of the SSEP with absent subsequent waves has also been observed in brain-dead patients [69]. Electroretinogram and electrocochleogram may also be considered before evaluating the VEP and BAEP in brain death [34].

CONCLUSION

Sensory evoked potential (EP) recording in critical head-injured patients is a useful tool to monitor the integrity of sensory input to the central nervous system. Short latency potentials reflect brainstem function, whereas middle and long latency potentials assess hemispheric function. A well defined correlation between clinical findings and EP recordings was noted. Sensory EPs are also valuable in monitoring anesthetized or paralyzed patients. Experience with deteriorating post-traumatic patients has shown EP monitoring to have significant clinical value. Localization of a brainstem lesion within several centimeters using brainstem auditory evoked potentials (BAEP) may be possible. Nevertheless, EPs test the functional rather than anatomic integrity of a specific tract. Sensory EP monitoring has proved to be an excellent predictor for outcome. The morbidity and mortality rates of post-traumatic coma are still high and there is a great need for frequent assessment and monitoring to improve the outcome of this challenging group of patients. More investigation remains to be done in head-injured patients as we find which sensory EP modalities correlate highest with neurological function and ultimate outcome.

REFERENCES

1. Achor LJ, Starr A. Audiology brainstem responses in the cat. II. Effects of lesions. Electroenceph Clin Neurophysiol, 1980, 48:174-190.

2. Adams JH, Mitchell DE, Graham DI, Doyle D. Diffuse brain damage of immediate impact type. Brain, 1977, 100:489-502.

3. Aguilar EA, Hall JW, Mackey-Hargadine J. Neuro-otologic evaluation of the patient with acute severe head injuries: correlations among physical findings, auditory evoked responses, and computerized tomography. Otolaryngol Head Neck Surg, 1986, 94:211-219.

4. Ahmed I. Brainstem auditory evoked potentials in transtentorial herniation. Clin Electroenceph, 1980, 11:34-37.

5. Alajouanine T, Scherrer J, Barbizet J, Calvet J, Verley R. Potentials evoques corticour chez des sujets atteints de troubles somesthetiques. Rev Neurol, 1958, 98:757-761.

6. Alani SM. Pattern-reversal visual evoked potentials in patients with hydrocephalus. J Neurosurg, 1985, 62:234-237.

7. Allen GW. Clinical implications of experiments on alteration of the labyrinthine fluid pressures. Otolaryng Clin No Am, 1983, 16:3-19.

8. Allen GW, Habibi M. The effect of increasing cerebrospinal fluid pressure upon the cochlear microphonics. Laryngoscope, 1962, 72:423-434.

9. Allison T, Hume AL. A comparative analysis of short-latency somatosensory evoked potentials in man, monkey, cat, and rat. Exp Neurol, 1981, 72:592-611.

10. American Electroencephalographic Society. Guidelines for clinical evoked potential studies. J Clin Neurophysiol, 1984, 1:3-53.

11. American Electroencephalographic Society. Guidelines for clinical evoked potential studies. J Clin Neurophysiol, 1986, 3(Suppl-1):43-92.

12. Anderson DC, Bundlie S, Rockswold GL. Multimodality evoked potentials in closed head trauma. Arch Neurol, 1984, 41:369-374.

13. Anziska BJ, Cracco RQ. Short latency somatosensory evoked potentials in patients with focal neurological disease. Electroenceph Clin Neurophysiol, 1980, 49:227-239.

14. Anziska BJ, Cracco RQ. Short latency SEPs to median nerve stimulation: comparison of recording methods and origin of components. Electroenceph Clin Neurophysiol, 1981, 52:531-539.

15. Asselman P, Chadwick DW, Marsiden CD. Visual evoked responses in the diagnosis and management of patients suspected of multiple sclerosis. Brain, 1975, 98:261-282.

16. Babel I, Stangos N, Korol S, Spiritus M. Ocular Electrophysiology: A clinical and experimental study of electroretinogram, electro-oculogram and visual evoked response. Stuttgart, George Thieme Publishers, 1977, pp 1-172.

17. Baker JB, Larson SJ, Sances A Jr, White PT. Evoked cortical potentials as an aid to the diagnosis of multiple sclerosis. Neurology, 1968, 18:286.

18. Barlas O, Gokay H, Turantan MI, et al. Adult aqueductal stenosis presenting with fluctuating hearing loss and vertigo. J Neurosurg, 1983, 59:703-705.

19. Benna P, Bergamasco B, Bianco C, Gilli M, Ferrero P, Pinessi L. Brainstem auditory evoked potentials in postconcussion syndrome. Ital J Neurol Sci, 1982a, 3(4):281-287.

20. Benna P, Gilli M, Ferrero P, Bergamasco B. Brainstem auditory evoked potentials in supratentorial tumors. Electroenceph Clin Neurophysiol, 1982b, 54:8-9.

21. Bergamasco B, Bergamini L, Mombelli AM, Mutani R. Longitudinal study of visual evoked potentials in different stages of coma. Electroenceph Clin Neurophysiol, 1966, 21:92.

22. Bergström L, Nystorm SHM. Visually evoked potentials in patients with brain lesions with or without disturbances of consciousness. Acta Neurol Scand, 1970, 46:562-572.

23. Boller F, Jacobson GP. Unilateral gunshot wound of the pons: Clinical, electrophysiologic and neuroradiographic correlates. Arch Neurol, 1980, 37:278-281.

24. Branston NM, Symon L, Crokard HA. Recovery of the cortical evoked response following temporal middle cerebral artery occlusion in baboons: Relation to local blood flow and PO2. Stroke, 1976, 7:151-157.

25. Brewer CC, Resnick DM. The value of BAEP in assessment of the comatose patients. in: Nodar RH, Barber C (eds), Evoked potentials II. Boston, London, Butterworth Publishers, 1984, pp 578-581.

26. Bricolo A, Faccioli F, Turazzi S, Pasut ML. EEG and evoked potentials in brainstem traumatic lesions. in: Villani R, Papo I, Giovanelli M, Gaini SM, Tomei G (eds), Advances in Neurotraumatology. Amsterdam-Oxford-Princeton, Exerpta Medica, 1983, pp 79-84.

27. Brown RH, Chiappa KH, Brooks EB. Brainstem auditory evoked responses in 22 patients with intrinsic brainstem lesions: Implications for clinical interpretations. Electroenceph Clin Neurophysiol, 1981, 51:38P.

28. Buchwald JS, Huang CM. Far-field acoustic response. Origins in the cat. Science, 1975, 189:382-384.

29. Butler RA, Honrubia V. Responses of cochlear potentials to changes in hydrostatic pressure. J Acoust Soc Am, 1963, 35:1188-1192.

30. Cant BR, Hume AL, Judson JA, Shaw NA. The assessment of severe head injury by short-latency somatosensory and brain-stem auditory evoked potentials. Electroenceph Clin Neurophysiol, 1986, 65:188-195.

31. Carlborg BIR, Farmer JC. Transmission of cerebrospinal fluid pressure via the cochlear aqueduct and endolymphatic sac. Am J Otolaryngol, 1983, 4:273-282.

32. Celesia G. Steady state and transient visual evoked potentials in clinical practice. Ann NY Acad Sci, 1982, 388:290-305.

33. Celesia GG, Soni VK, Rhode WS. Visual evoked spectrum array and interhemispheric variations. Arch Neurol, 1978, 35:678-682.

34. Chiappa KH. Evoked Potentials in Clinical Medicine, 2nd edition. Chiappa KH (ed), New York, Raven Press, 1990.

35. Chiappa KH. Interpretation of abnormal short-latency somatosensory evoked potentials. In: Halliday AM, Butler SR, Paul R (eds), A Textbook of Clinical Neurophysiology. New York, John Wiley and Sons, 1987, pp 343-381.

36. Chiappa KH, Choi SK, Young RR. Short latency somatosensory evoked potentials following median nerve stimulation in patients with neurological lesions. In: Desmedt JE (ed), Clinical uses of cerebral, brainstem, and spinal somatosensory evoked potentials. Prog Clin Neurophysiol. Basel, Karger, 1980, pp 264-281.

37. Chiappa RH, Gladstone KJ, Young RR. Brain stem auditory evoked responses: studies of waveform variations in 50 normal human subjects. Arch Neurol, 1979, 36:81-87.

38. Chiappa RH, Young RR, Goldie WD. Origins of the components of human short-latency somatosensory evoked responses (SER). Neurology, 1979, 29:598.

39. Clague B, Lorig RJ, Weiss MH, Nulsen FE, Brodkey JS. Comparative effects of increased intracranial pressure upon cerebral oxygenation, cortical evoked potential and brain survival. Stroke (Abstract), 1973, 4:346.

40. Clark JB, Bellegarrique RB, Salcman M. Gunshot wound to the pons with functional neuroanatomical and electrophysiological correlation. Neurosurg, 1985, 16:607-611.

41. Coats AC. Human auditory nerve action potentials and brainstem evoked response. Latency-intensity functions in detection of cochlear and retrocochlear pathology. Arch Otolaryngol, 1978, 104:709-717.

42. Coats AC, Martin JL. Human auditory nerve action potentials and brainstem evoked responses. Effects of audiogram shape and lesion location. Arch Otolaryngol, 1977, 103:605-622.

43. Cracco RQ, Cracco JB. Somatosensory evoked potential in man: Far field potentials. Electroenceph Clin Neurophysiol, 1976, 41:460-466.

44. Creutzfeld OD, Kuhnt U. The visual evoked potential: Physiological developmental and clinical aspects. Electroenceph Clin Neurophysiol, 1967 (suppl), 26:29-41.

45. De La Torre JC, Trimple JL, Beard RT, Hanlon K, Surgeon TW. Somatosensory evoked potentials for the prognosis of coma in humans. Exp Neurol, 1978, 60:304-317.

46. Desmedt JE. Relevance of somatosensory evoked potential measures for tropical diagnosis of brainstem lesions. In: Kunze K, Zangemeister WH, Arlt A (eds), Clinical Problems of Brainstem Disorders. New York, Georg Thieme Verlag Stuttgart, 1986, pp 82-88.

47. Despland PA. Evoked response audiometry. In: Halliday AM, Butler SR, Paul R (eds), A Textbook of Clinical Neurophysiology. New York, John Wiley and Sons, 1987, pp 399-414.

48. Despland P, Galambos K. Use of auditory brainstem responses by premature and newborn infants. Neuropediatrics, 1980, 11:99-107.

49. Deutsch E, Sohmer H, Weidenfeld J, Zelic S, Chowers I. Auditory nerve-brain stem evoked potentials and EEG during severe hypoglycemia. Electroenceph Clin Neurophysiol, 1983, 55:714-716.

50. de Vlieger M, Sadikoglu S, Van Eigndhoven JHM. Visual evoked potentials, auditory evoked potentials and EEG in shunted hydrocephalic children. Neuropediatrics, 1981, 12:55-61.

51. Ducati A, Parmigiani F, Antonelli A, Villani R. Early evaluation of prognosis using BAERs in patients with posttraumatic disorders of consciousness. in: Villani R, Papo I, Giovanelli M, Gaini SM, Tomei G (eds), Advances in Neurotraumatology. Amsterdam-Oxford-Princeton, Exerpta Medica, 1983, pp 214-216.

52. Edwards CG, Durieux-Smith A, Picton TW. Auditory brainstem response audiometry in neonatal hydrocephalus. J Otolaryngol, 1985, 14(Suppl):40-46.

53. Eggermont JJ, Don M. Mechanisms of central conduction time prolongation in brain-stem auditory evoked potentials. Arch Neurol, 1986, 43:116-120.

54. Ehle A, Sklar F. Visual evoked potentials in infants with hydrocephalus. Neurology, 1979, 29:1541-1544.

55. Eisen A, Aminoff MJ. Somatosensory evoked potentials. In: Aminoff MJ (ed), Electrodiagnosis in Clinical Neurology. Churchill Livingstone, 1986, pp 535-573.

56. Engel RC. Abnormal electroencephalograms in the neonatal period. Springfield IL, Charles C Thomas, 1975, pp 106-116.

57. Facco E, Martini A, Zuccarello M, Agnoletto M, Giron GP. Is the auditory brain-stem response (ABR) effective in the assessment of post-traumatic coma? Electroenceph Clin Neurophysiol, 1985, 62:332-337.

58. Feldman MR. Effects of increased cerebrospinal fluid pressure on CM response. J Speech Hearing Research, 1968, 11:18-32.

59. Fichsel H. Diagnosis of hydrocephalus. Changes in visual evoked potentials in children with progressive hydrocephalus internus. Fortschr Med (Ger), 1976, 94:1141-1142.

60. Foit A, Larson B, Hattori S, Skinhoj E, Lassen NA. Cortical activation during somatosensory stimulation and voluntary movement in man: A regional cerebral blood flow study. Electroenceph Clin Neurophysiol, 1980, 50:426-436.

61. Foltz EL, Blanks JP, McPherson DL. Hydrocephalus: Increased intracranial pressure and brainstem auditory evoked responses in the hydrocephalic rabbits. Neurosurgery, 1987, 20:211-217.

62. Gennarelli TA. Cerebral concussion and diffuse brain injuries. in: Cooper P (ed), Head Injury 2nd ed, Baltimore, Williams & Wilkins, 1987, pp 108-124.

63. Ghaly RF, Stone JL, Subramanian KS, Roccaforte P, Hughes JR. Modified auditory brainstem response (MABR). Part II: Studies in patients with intracranial lesions. Clin Electroenceph, 1988, 19:95-107.

64. Giblin DR. Somatosensory evoked potentials in healthy subjects and in patients with lesions of the nervous system. Ann NY Acad Sci, 1964, 112:93-142.

65. Gibson WPR. Electrocochleography. In: Halliday AM (ed), Evoked Potentials in Clinical Testing, London, Churchill Livingstone, 1982, pp 283-311.

66. Glattke TJ. Short-Latency Auditory Evoked Potentials. Baltimore, University Park Press, 1983, 141 pps.

67. Glover JL, Worth RM, Bendick PJ, et al. Evoked responses in the diagnosis of thoracic outlet syndrome. Surgery, 1981, 89:89.

68. Goitein KJ, Fainmesse P, Sohmer H. The relationship between cerebral perfusion pressure and auditory nerve brain stem evoked response — Diagnostic and prognostic implications. In: Ishii S, Nagai H, Brock M (eds), Intracranial Pressure V. Berlin-Heidelberg, Springer Verlag, 1983, pp 468-473.

69. Goldie WD, Chiappa KH, Young RR, Brooks EB. Brain stem auditory and short latency somatosensory evoked responses in brain death. Neurology, 1981, 31:248-256.

70. Greenberg RP, Mayer DJ, Becker DP, Miller JD. Evaluation of brain function in severe human head trauma with multimodality evoked potentials. Part I: Evoked brain-injury potentials, methods, and analysis. J Neurosurg, 1977, 47:150-162.

71. Greenberg RP, Becker DP, Miller JD, Mayer DJ. Evaluation of brain function in severe human head trauma with multimodality evoked potentials. Part 2: Localization of brain dysfunction and correlation with posttraumatic neurological conditions. J Neurosurg, 1977, 47:163-177.

72. Greenberg RP, Ducker TB. Evoked potentials in the clinical neurosciences. J Neurosurg, 1982, 56:1-18.

73. Greenberg RP, Newlon PG, Hyatt MS, Narayan RK, Becker DP. Prognostic implications of early multimodality evoked potentials in severely head-injured patients. A prospective study. J Neurosurg, 1981, 55:227-236.

74. Grossman RG, Turner JW, Miller JD, Rowan JO. The relationship between cortical electrical activity, cerebral perfusion pressure and cerebral blood flow during increased intracranial pressure. Stroke, 1973 (Abstract), 4:346.

75. Grundy BL. Evoked potential monitoring. In: Blitt CO (ed), Monitoring in Anesthesia and Critical Care Medicine. Churchill Livingstone, 1985, pp 345-411.

76. Gupta NK, Verma NP, Guidice MA, Kooi KA. Visual evoked response in head trauma: pattern-shift stimulus. Neurology, 1986, 36:578-581.

77. Guthkelch AN, Sclabassi RJ, Hirsch RP, Vries JK. Visual evoked potentials in hydrocephalus: relationship to head size, shunting, and mental development. Neurosurg, 1984, 14:283-286.

78. Guthkelch AN, Sclabassi RJ, Vries JK. Changes in the visual evoked potentials of hydrocephalic children. Neurosurgery, 1982, 11:599-602.

79. Hall JW. Auditory brainstem response spectral content in comatose head-injured patients. Ear and Hearing, 1986, 7:383-389.

80. Hall JW, Brown DP, Mackey-Hargadine JR. Pediatric application of serial auditory brain stem and middle-latency evoked response recordings. Int J Ped Otorhinolaryngol, 1985, 9:201-218.

81. Hall JW, Huangfu M, Gennarelli TA. Auditory function in acute severe head injury. Laryngoscope, 1982, 92:883-890.

82. Hall JW, Huangfu M, Gennarelli TA, Dolinskas CA, Olson K, Berry GA. Auditory evoked responses, impedance measures, and diagnostic speech audiometry in severe head injury. Otolaryngol Head Neck Surg, 1983, 91:50-60.

83. Hall JW, Huangfu M, Gennarelli TA, Kimmelman CP, Dolinskas CA. Auditory brainstem abnormalities in experimental and clinical acute severe head injury. Acad Ophthalmology and Otolaryngol, 1983, 36:83-88.

84. Hall JW III, Mackey-Hargadine J. Auditory evoked responses in severe head injury. In: Semin Hearing, 1984, 5: 313-336.

85. Hall JW, Morgan SH, Mackey-Hargadine J, Aguilar EA, Jahrsdoerfer RA. Neurotologic applications of simultaneous multichannel auditory evoked response recordings. Laryngoscope, 1984, 94:883-889.

86. Halliday AM. Evoked Potentials in Clinical Testing. Churchill Livingstone, 1982.
87. Halliday AM, Halliday E, Kriss A, et al. The pattern evoked potentials in compression of the anterior visual pathways. Brain, 1976, 99:357-374.
88. Halliday AM, Mushin J. The visual evoked potential in neuroophthalmology. Int Ophthalmol Clin, 1980, 20:155-185.
89. Hammond EJ, Wilder BJ, Goodman IJ, Hunter SB. Auditory brain stem potentials with unilateral pontine hemorrhage. Arch Neurol, 1985, 42:767-768.
90. Hashimoto I. Somatosensory evoked potentials from the human brainstem: origins of short-latency potentials. Electroenceph Clin Neurophysiol, 1984, 57:221-227.
91. Hashimoto I, Ishiyama Y, Tozuka G. Bilaterally recorded brain stem auditory evoked responses, their asymmetric abnormalities and lesions of the brain stem. Arch Neurol, 1979, 36:161-167.
92. Hecox KE, Cone B, Blaw ME. Brainstem auditory evoked response in the diagnosis of pediatric neurologic diseases. Neurology, 1981, 31:832-840.
93. Hecox KE, Galambos R. Brainstem auditory evoked responses in human infants and adults. Arch Otolaryngol, 1974, 99:30-33.
94. Hillayard SA, Picton TW, Regan D. Sensation, perception, and attention. Analysis using ERPs. In: Callaway E, Tueting P, and Koslow SH (eds), Event-Related Brain Potentials in Man. New York, Academic Press, 1978, pp 223-321.
95. Hughes JR, Fino J. Usefulness of piezoelectric earphones in recording the brainstem auditory evoked potentials: A new early deflection. Electroenceph Clin Neurophysiol, 1980, 48:357-360.
96. Hume AL, Cant BR. Pattern visual evoked potentials in the diagnosis of multiple sclerosis and other disorders. Proc Austr Assoc Neurol, 1976, 13:7-13.
97. Hume AL, Cant BR. Conduction time in central somatosensory pathways in man. Electroenceph Clin Neurophysiol, 1978, 45:361-75.
98. Hume AL, Cant BR. Central somatosensory conduction after head injury. Ann Neurol, 1981, 10:411-419.
99. Humphery PRD, Moseley IF, Ross Russell RW. Visual field defects in obstructive hydrocephalus. J Neurol Neurosurg Psychiat, 1982, 45:591-597.
100. Humphries KN, Ashcroft PB, Douek EE. Extra-tympanic electrocochleography. Acta Otolaryngol, 1977, 83:303-309.
101. Jennett WB, Stern WE. Tentorial herniation, the midbrain and the pupil. Experimental studies in brain compression. J Neurosurg, 1966, 17:598-609.
102. Jewett DL. Volume conducted potentials in response to auditory stimuli as detected by averaging in the cat. Electroenceph Clin Neurophysiol, 1970, 28:609-618.
103. Jones SJ. Short latency potentials recorded from the neck and scalp following median nerve stimulation in man. Electroenceph Clin Neurophysiol, 1977, 43:853-863.
104. Jones SJ. Investigation of brachial plexus traction lesions by peripheral and spinal somatosensory evoked potentials. J Neurol Neurosurg Psychiat, 1979, 42:107-116.
105. Kaga K, Nagai T, Takamori A, Marsh RR. Auditory short, middle, and long latency responses in acutely comatose patients. Laryngoscope (St. Louis), 1985, 95:321-325.
106. Karnaze DS. Marshall LF, McCarthy CS, Klauber MR, Bickford RG. Localizing and prognostic value of auditory evoked responses in coma after closed head injury. Neurology, 1982, 32:299-302.
107. Karnaze DS, Weiner JM, Marshall LF. Auditory evoked potentials in coma after closed head injury: A clinical-neurophysiologic coma scale for predicting outcome. Neurology, 1985, 35:1122-1126.
108. Kawahara N, Sasaki M, Mii K, Tsuzuki M, Takakura K. Sequential changes of auditory brain stem responses in relation to intracranial and cerebral perfusion pressure, and initiation of secondary brain stem damage. Acta Neurochir (Wien), 1989, 100:142-149

109. Keith RW, Jabre AF, Heerse KL. Auditory brainstem response testing in the surgical intensive care unit. Semin Hearing, 1983, 4:385-389.
110. Kerth JD, Allen GW. Comparison of the perilymphatic and cerebrospinal fluid pressures. Arch Otolaryngol, 1963, 77:581-585.
111. Kirkham TH, Coupland SG. Abnormal electroretinogram and visual evoked potentials in chronic papilledema using time difference analysis. Can J Neurol Sci, 1981, 8:243-248.
112. Kjaer M. Localizing brain stem lesions with brain stem auditory evoked potentials. Acta Neurol Scand, 1980, 61:265-274.
113. Klug N. Brainstem auditory evoked potentials in syndromes of decerebration, the bulbar syndrome and in central death. J Neurol, 1982, 227:219-228.
114. Klug N, Csecsei G, Rap ZM. Evoked potentials and blink reflex in acute midbrain syndromes. Clinical and experimental findings. In: Villani R, Papo I, Giovanelli M, Gaini SM, Tomei G (eds), Advances in Neurotraumatology. Amsterdam-Oxford-Princeton, Exerpta Medica, 1983, pp 207-209.
115. Kraus N, Ozdamar O, Heydemann PT, Stein LO, Reed NL. Auditory brain-stem responses in hydrocephalic patients. Electroenceph Clin Neurophysiol, 1984, 59:310-317.
116. Kudo Y, Yamadori A. Somatosensory evoked potentials in patients with thalamic lesions. J Neurol, 1985, 232:61-66.
117. Kuroiwa Y, Celesia GG. Visual evoked potentials with hemifield pattern stimulation. their use in the diagnosis of retrochiasmatic lesions. Arch Neurol, 1981, 38:86-90.
118. Laget P, Mamo H, Houndart R. De l'interet des potentiels evoques somesthetiques dans l'etude des lesions du lobe parietal de l'homme, etude des preliminaire. Neurochir, 1967, 13:841-853.
119. Larson SJ, Sances A, Ackmann JJ, Reigel DH. Non invasive evaluation of head trauma patients. Surgery, 1973, 74:34-40.
120. Larson SJ, Sances A Jr, Baker JB. Evoked cortical potentials in patients with stroke. Circulation, 1966, 23(Suppl 2):15-19.
121. Lastimosa ACB, Bass NH, Stanback K, Norvell EE. Lumbar spinal cord and early cortical evoked potentials after tibial nerve stimulation: Effects of stature on normative data. Electroenceph Clin Neurophysiol, 1982, 54:499-507.
122. Legouix JP. Changes in the cochlear microphonic of the guinea pig produced by mechanical factors in the inner ear. J Acoust Soc Am, 1962, 34:1504-1508.
123. Lev A, Sohmer H. Sources of averaged neural responses recorded in animal and human subjects during cochlear audiometry (electrocochleography). Archiv Klin, 1972, 201:79-90.
124. Liberson WT. Study of evoked potentials in aphasics. Amer J Phys Med, 1966, 45:135-142.
125. Lindsay KW, Carlin J, Kennedy I, Fry J, McInnes A, Teasdale GM. Evoked potentials in severe head injury—analysis and relation to outcome. J Neurol Neurosurg Psychiat, 1981, 44:796-802.
126. Lindsay KW, Pasaoglu A, Hirst D, Allardyce G, Kennedy I, Teasdale G. Somatosensory and auditory brain stem conduction after head injury: A comparison with clinical features in prediction of outcome. Neurosurg, 1990, 26:278-285.
127. Lueders H, Andrish J, Gurd A, Weiker G, Klem G. Origin of far-field subcortical potentials evoked by stimulation of the posterior tibial nerve. Electroenceph Clin Neurophysiol, 1981, 52:336-344.
128. Lueders H, Lesser R, Hahn J, Little J, Klem G. Subcortical somatosensory evoked potentials to median nerve stimulation. Brain, 1983, 106:341-372.
129. Lutschg J, Pfenninger J, Ludin HP, Vassella F. Brain stem auditory evoked potentials and early somatosensory evoked potentials in neurointensively treated comatose children. Am J Dis Child, 1983, 137:421-426.
130. Mackey-Hargadine J, Hall JW. Rationale for neuromonitoring in intensive care unit. Presented at the IEEE/EMBS 8th Annual conference, Ft Worth TX, November 7-10, 1986.

131. Mackey-Hargadine J, Hall JW. Sensory evoked responses in head injury. J Am Paralysis Assoc, 1985, 2:187-206.

132. Mackay AR, Hosobuchi Y, Williston JS, Jewett D. Brain stem auditory evoked responses and brain stem compression. Neurosurg, 1980, 6:632-638.

133. Marcus EM, Girouard R, Stone B. Short-latency evoked responses in evaluation of comatose patients. Trans Am Neurol Assoc, 1980, 105:207-211.

134. Marcus EM, Stone B. Short-latency median nerve somatosensory evoked potentials in coma: Relationship to BAEP, etiology, age, and outcome. In: Nodar RH, Barber D (eds), Evoked Potentials II. Boston, London, Butterworth Publishers, 1984, pp 609-623.

135. Matsuura S, Kuno M, Nakamura T. Intracranial pressure and auditory evoked responses of the cat. Acta Otolaryngol (Stokh), 1986, 102:12-19.

136. Mauguiere F, Courjon J, Schott B. Dissociation of early SEP components in unilateral traumatic section of the lower medulla. Ann Neurol, 1983, 13:309-313.

137. Mauguiere F, Desmedt JE, Courjon J. Neural generators of N18 and N14 far-field somatosensory evoked potentials: patients with lesion of thalamus or thalamocortical radiations. Electroenceph Clin Neurophysiol, 1983, 56:283-292.

138. McCabe BR, Wolsk D. Experimental inner ear pressure changes. Ann Otorhinolaryngol, 1961, 70:541-555.

139. McInnes A. Evoked potentials in hydrocephalus. Electroenceph Clin Neurophysiol, 1980 (Abstract), 50:233P-234P.

140. McPherson D, Blanks J, Foltz E. Intracranial pressure effects on auditory evoked responses in the rabbit: preliminary report. Neurosurg, 1986, 14:161-166.

141. McSherry JW, Walters CL. Acute visual evoked potential changes in hydrocephalus. Electroenceph Clin Neurophysiol, 1982, 53:331-333.

142. Mjoen S, Nordby HK, Torvik A. Auditory evoked brainstem responses (ABR) in coma due to severe head trauma. Acta Otolaryngol, 1983, 95:131-138.

143. Monnier M. Visual occipital potentials. Ophthalmologica, 1974, 169:160-175.

144. Nagao S, Kuyama H, Honma Y, Momma F, Nishiura T, Murota T, Suga M, Tanimoto T, Kawauchi M, Nishimoto A. Prediction and evaluation of brainstem function by auditory brainstem responses in patients with uncal herniation. Surg Neurol, 1987, 27:81-86.

145. Nagao S, Roccaforte P, Moody RA. Acute intracranial hypertension and auditory brain-stem responses. Part I: Changes in the auditory brain-stem and somatosensory evoked responses in intracranial hypertension in cats. J Neurosurg, 1979, 51:669-676.

146. Nagao S, Roccaforte P, Moody RA. Acute intracranial hypertension and auditory brain-stem responses. Part 2: The effects of brain-stem movement on the auditory brain-stem responses due to transtentorial herniation. J Neurosurg, 1979, 51:846-851.

147. Nagao S, Roccaforte P, Moody RA. Acute intracranial hypertension and auditory brain-stem responses. Part 3: The effects of posterior fossa mass lesions on brain-stem function. J Neurosurg, 1980, 52:351-358.

148. Nagao S, Sumani N, Tsutsui T, Honma Y, Monna F, Nishiura T, Nishimoto A. Diagnosis of uncal herniation by auditory brain-stem response. Neurol Med Chir (Tokyo), 1984, 24:396-400.

149. Nagao S, Sunami N, Tsutsui T, Honma Y, Fujimoto S, Ohmoto T, Nishimoto A. Serial observations of brain stem function in acute intracranial hypertension by auditory brain stem responses — A clinical study. In: Ishii S, Nagai H, Brock M (eds), Intracranial Pressure V. Berlin-Heidelberg, Springer Verlag, 1983, pp 474-479.

150. Nagao S, Sunami N, Tsutsui T, Honma Y, Doi A, Nishimoto A. Serial observations of brain stem function by auditory brain stem responses in central transtentorial herniation. Surg Neurol, 1982, 17:355-357.

151. Nagao S, Sunami N, Tsutsui T, Honma Y, Mamma F, Nishiura T, Nishimoto A. Acute intracranial hypertension and brainstem blood flow. J Neurosurg, 1984, 60:566-571.

152. Nagata K, Tazawa T, Mizukami M, Araki G. Application of brainstem auditory evoked potentials to evaluation of cerebral herniation. In: Nodar RH, Barber C (eds), Evoked Potentials II. Boston, London, Butterworth Publishers, 1984, pp 183-193.

153. Nakanishi T, Tamaki M, Arasaki K, Kudo N. Origins of the scalp-recorded somatosensory far field potentials in man and cat. Electroenceph Clin Neurophysiol, 1982, 36(Suppl):336-348.

154. Narayan RK, Greenberg RP, Miller JD, Enas GG, Choi SC, Kishore PRS, Selhorst JB, Lutz HA, Becker DP. Improved confidence of outcome prediction in severe head injury. A comparative analysis of the clinical examination, multimodality evoked potentials, CT scanning, and intracranial pressure. J Neurosurg, 1981, 54:751-762.

155. Narayan RK, Kishore PR, Becker DP, Ward JD, Enas GG, Greenberg RP, Da Silva AD, Lipper MH, Choi SC, Mayhall CG, Lutz HA, Young HF. Intracranial pressure to monitor or not to monitor? A review of our experience with severe head injury. J Neurosurg, 1981, 55:650-659.

156. Newlon PG, Greenberg RP. Evoked potentials in severe head injury. J Trauma, 1984, 24:61-66.

157. Newlon PG, Greenberg RP, Hyatt MS, Enas GG, Becker DP. The dynamics of neuronal dysfunction and recovery following severe head injury assessed with serial multimodality evoked potentials. J Neurosurg, 1982, 57:168-177.

158. Nodar RH, Hahn J, Levine HL. Brain stem auditory evoked potentials in determining site of lesion of brain stem gliomas in children. Laryngoscope (St. Louis), 1980, 90:258-265.

159. Noel P, Desmedt JE. Cerebral and far-field somatosensory evoked potentials in neurological disorders involving the cervical spinal cord, brainstem, thalamus, and cortex. In: Desmedt JE, Karger KS (eds), Clinical uses of cerebral, brainstem and spinal somatosensory evoked potentials. Progress in Clinical Neurophysiology, Vol 7. Basel, Karger, 1980, pp 205-230.

160. Oh, SJ, Kubat T, Kuba T, Soyer, A, Choi S, Bonikowski FP, Vitek JT. Lateralization of brainstem lesions by brainstem auditory evoked potentials. Neurology, 1981, 31:14-18.

161. Oken BS, Chiappa RH. Electroencephalography and evoked potentials in head trauma. In: Becker DP, Povlishock JT (eds), Central Nervous System Trauma — Status Report. Washington, NIH, 1985, 177-185.

162. Olbrich HM, Nau HE, Lodemann E, Zerbin D, Schmit-Neuerburg KP. Evoked potential assessment of mental function during recovery from severe head injury. Surg Neurol, 1986, 26:112-118.

163. Ommaya AK, Gennarelli T. Cerebral concussion and traumatic unconsciousness — correlation of experimental and clinical observations on blunt head injuries. Brain, 1974, 97:633-654.

164. Ommaya AK, Gennarelli T. A physiopathologic basis for noninvasive diagnosis and prognosis of head injury severity. In: McLaurin RL (ed), Head Injuries. New York, Grune and Stratton, 1976, pp 49-75.

165. Onofrj M, Bodis-Wollner I, Mylin L. Visual evoked potential latencies in papilledema and hydrocephalus. Neuroophthalmology, 1981, 2:85-92.

166. Ottaviani F, Almadori G, Calderazzo AB, Frenguelli A, Paludetti G. Auditory brain stem (ABRs) and middle-latency auditory responses (MLRs) in the prognosis of severely head-injured patients. Electroenceph Clin Neurophysiol, 1986, 65:196-202.

167. Papanicolaou AC, Levin HS, Eisenberg HM, Moore BD, Goethe KE, High WN Jr. Evoked potential correlates of posttraumatic amnesia after closed head injury. Neurosurg, 1984, 14:676-678.

168. Papanicolaou AC, Loring DW, Eisenberg HM, Raz N, Contreras FL. Auditory brain stem evoked responses in comatose head-injured patients. Neurosurg, 1986, 18:173-175.

169. Perot PL. Evoked potentials assessment of patients with neural trauma. In: McLaurin RL (ed), Head Injuries. New York, Grune and Stratton, 1976, pp 77-79.

170. Picton TW, Woods DL, Baribeau-Braun J, et al. Evoked potential audiometry. J Otolaryngology, 1977, 6:90-118.

171. Pfurtscheller G, Schwarz G, Gravenstein N. Clinical relevance of long-latency SEPs and VEPs during coma and emergence from coma. Electroenceph Clin Neurophysiol, 1985, 62:88-98.

172. Pratt H, Ben-David Y, Peled R, Podoshin L, Scharf B. Auditory brainstem evoked potentials: Clinical promise of increasing stimulus rate. Electroenceph Clin Neurophysiol, 1981, 51:80-90.

173. Prugger M, Rumpl E, Gerstenbrand F, Hackl JM. Central somatosensory conduction time and early SEP components in posttraumatic coma. In: Villani R, Papo I, Giovanelli M, Gaini SM, Tomei G (eds), Advances in Neurotraumatology. Amsterdam-Oxford-Princeton, Exerpta Medica, 1983, pp 210-213.

174. Raimondi AJ, Hirschauer J. Head Injury in the infant and toddler: coma scoring and outcome scale. In: Villani R, Papo I, Giovanelli M, Gaini SM, Tomei G (eds), Advances in Neurotraumatology. Amsterdam-Oxford-Princeton, Exerpta Medica, 1983, pp 99-106.

175. Rappaport M, Hopkins R, Hall K, Belleza T, Berrol S, Reynolds G. Evoked brain potentials and disability in brain damaged patients. Arch Phys Med Rehabil, 1977, 58:333-338.

176. Raudzens P, Scharber R, Erspamer R. Intracranial pressure effects on brainstem potentials. Anesthesiology, 1979, 51:S40.

177. Robinson F. Influence of increased intracranial pressure on evoked responses to sensory stimulation. Electroenceph Clin Neurophysiol, 1967 (Abstract), 23:96.

178. Robinson K, Rudge P. Centrally generated auditory potentials. In Halliday AM (ed), Evoked Potentials in Clinical Testing. London, Churchill Livingstone, 1982, pp 345-372.

179. Ropper RH, Miller DC. Acute traumatic midbrain hemorrhage. Ann Neurol, 1985, 18:80-86.

180. Rosenberg C, Wogensen K, Starr A. Auditory brain-stem and middle and long-latency evoked potentials in coma. Arch Neurol, 1984, 41:835-838.

181. Rossini P, Gambi D, Di Rocco C, et al. Study of visually evoked potentials in children with hydrocephalus. Riv Neurol (Ital), 1978, 48:594-598.

182. Rouher F, Plane C, Sole P. Interet des potentiels evoques visuels dans les affections du nerf optique. Arch Ophthalmol (Paris), 1969, 29:555-564.

183. Rumpl E, Prugger M, Gerstenbrand F, Hackl JM, Paliua A. Central somatosensory conduction time and short latency somatosensory evoked potentials in post-traumatic coma. Electroenceph Clin Neurophysiol, 1983, 56:583-596.

184. Saxena RK, Tandon PN, Sinha A, et al. Auditory functions in raised intracranial pressure. Acta Otolaryngol, 1969, 68:402-410.

185. Scarpino O, Mauro AM, Signorino M, Guidi M, Brunellini P, Testasecca D. Prognostic value of brainstem auditory evoked potentials in traumatic coma. In: Villani R, Papo I, Giovanelli M, Gaini SM, Tomei G (eds), Advances in Neurotraumatology. Amsterdam-Oxford-Princeton, Exerpta Medica, 1983, pp 224-226.

186. Scherg M, Cramon DV, Elton M. Brain stem auditory evoked potentials in post-comatose patients after severe closed head trauma. J Neurology, 1984, 231:1-5.

187. Seals M, Rossiter VS, Weinstein ME. Brain stem auditory evoked responses in patients comatose as a result of blunt head trauma. J Trauma, 1979, 19:347-352.

188. Seelig JM, Greenberg RP, Becker DP, Miller JD, Choi SC. Reversible brain-stem dysfunction following acute traumatic subdural hematoma. A clinical and electrophysiological study. J Neurosurg, 1981, 55:516-523.

189. Sklar FH, Ehle AL, Clark WK. Visual evoked potentials: A noninvasive technique to monitor patients with shunted hydrocephalus. Neurosurg, 1979, 4:529-534.

190. Skondras S, Kountouris D, Skondra M. BAEP abnormality: indicator of increased intracranial pressure? Electromyogr Clin Neurophysiol, 1986, 26:107-115.

191. Sohmer H. Neurologic disorders. In: Moore EJ (ed), Bases of Auditory Brainstem Evoked Responses. New York, Grune and Stratton, 1983, pp 317-341.

192. Sohmer H, Gafni M, Chisin R. Auditory nerve and brain stem responses, comparison in awake and unconscious subject. Arch Neurol, 1978, 35:228-230.

193. Sohmer H, Gafni M, Goitein K, Feinmesser P. Auditory nerve-brain stem evoked potentials in cats during manipulation of the cerebral perfusion pressure. Electroenceph Clin Neurophysiol, 1983, 55:198-202.

194. Sohmer H, Gafni M, Havatselet G. Persistence of auditory nerve response and absence of brain-stem response in severe cerebral ischemia. Electroenceph Clin Neurophysiol, 1984, 58:65-72.

195. Sohmer H, Feinmesser M, Szabo G. Sources of electrocochleographic responses as studied in patients with brain damage. Electroenceph Clin Neurophysiol, 1974, 37:663-669.

196. Starr A. Auditory brain stem responses in brain death. Brain, 1976, 99:543-554.

197. Starr A. Auditory brainstem potentials: Their theory in practice in evaluating neural function. in: Halliday AM, Butler SR, Paul R (eds), A Textbook of Clinical Neurophysiology. New York, John Wiley and Sons, 1987, pp 383-398.

198. Starr A, Achor LJ. Auditory brain stem responses in neurological disease. Arch Neurol, 1975, 32:761-768.

199. Starr A, Hamilton AE. Correlation between confirmed sites of neurological lesions and abnormalities of far-field auditory brain stem responses. Electroenceph Clin Neurophysiol, 1976, 41:595-608.

200. Starr A, Sohmer H, Celesia GG. Some applications of evoked potentials in patients with neurological and sensory impairment. In: Callaway E, Tueting P, Koslow SH (eds), Event-Related Brain Potentials in Man. New York, Academic Press, 1978.

201. Stockard JJ, Rossiter VS. Clinical and pathologic correlates of brain stem auditory responses abnormalities. Neurology, 1977, 27:316-325.

202. Stockard JJ, Stockard JE, Sharbrough FW. Brainstem auditory evoked potentials in neurology: Methodology, interpretation, and clinical application. In: Aminoff MJ (ed), Electrodiagnosis in Clinical Neurology. New York, Churchill Livingstone, 1986, pp 467-503.

203. Stone JL, Bouffard A, Morris R, Hovsepian W, Meyers HL. Clinical and electrophysiologic recovery in Arnold-Chiari malformation. Surg Neurol, 1983, 20:313-317.

204. Stone JL, Ghaly RF, Subramanian KS, Roccaforte P, Hughes JR. Modified auditory brainstem responses (MABR): Part 1: Rationale and normative study. Clin Electroenceph, 1987, 18:218-226.

205. Stone JL, Ghaly RF, Subramanian KS, Roccaforte P, Kane J. Transtentorial brain herniation in the monkey: Analysis of brainstem auditory and somatosensory evoked potentials. Neurosurg, 1990, 26:26-31.

206. Sutton LN, Cho BK, Jaggi J, Joseph PM, Bruce DA. Effects of hydrocephalus and increased intracranial pressure on auditory and somatosensory evoked responses. Neurosurg, 1986, 18:756-761.

207. Symon L, Wang A. Clinical application of somatosensory evoked potentials as a monitor of brain ischemia. In: Nodar RH, Barber C (eds), Evoked Potentials II. Boston London, Butterworth Publishers, 1984, pp 572-577.

208. Teasdale G, Jennett B. Assessment of coma and impaired consciousness. A practical scale. Lancet, 1974, 2:81-84.

209. Thornton ARD, Hawkes CH. Neurological applications of surface-recorded electrocochleography. J Neurol Neurosurg Psychiat, 1976, 39:586-592.

210. Trojaborg W, Jorgensen EO. Evoked cortical potentials in patients with isoelectric EEGs. Electroenceph Clin Neurophysiol, 1973, 35:301-309.

211. Tsubokawa T, Kondo T, Higashi H, Takeuchi T, Goto T, Sugawara T, Hayashi N, Moriyasu N. Operative indications of large decompressive craniectomy for cerebral contusion with subdural hematoma. Neurol Med Chir (Tokyo), 1979, 19:771-780.

212. Tsubokawa T, Nishimoto H, Yamamoto T, Kitamura M, Katayama Y, Moriyasu N. Assessment of brainstem damage by the auditory brainstem response in acute severe head injury. J Neurol Neurosurg Psychiat, 1980, 43:1005-1011.
213. Uziel A, Benezech J. Auditory brain-stem responses in comatose patients. Relationship with brain-stem reflexes and levels of coma. Electroenceph Clin Neurophysiol, 1978, 45:515-524.
214. Vaughan HG, Katzman R. Evoked response in visual disorders. Ann NY Acad Sci, 1964, 112:305-319.
215. Vickova M. Visual evoked potentials in intracranial hypertension. Sb Ved Pr Lek Fak Karlovy Univ, 1974, 17(Suppl-4):283-288.
216. Walser H, Emre M, Janzer R. Somatosensory evoked potentials in comatose patients: correlation with outcome and neuropathological findings. J Neurol, 1986, 233:34-40.
217. Williamson PD, Goff WR, Allison T. Somatosensory evoked responses in patients with unilateral cerebral lesions. Electroenceph Clin Neurophysiol, 1970, 28:566-575.
218. Witzman A. Changes of somatosensory evoked potentials with increase of intracranial pressure in the rat's brain. Electroenceph Clin Neurophysiol, 1990, 77:59-67.
219. Woods DL, Kwee I, Clayworth CC, Kramer JH, Nakada T. Sensory and cognitive evoked potentials in a case of congenital hydrocephalus. Electroenceph Clin Neurophysiol, 1987, 68:202-208.
220. Yagi T, Baba S. Evaluation of the brain stem function by the auditory brain stem response and the caloric vestibular reaction in comatose patient. Arch Otolaryngol, 1983, 238:33-43.
221. York DH. Correlation between a unilateral midbrain-pontine lesion and abnormalities of brain stem auditory evoked potential. Electroenceph Clin Neurophysiol, 1986, 65:282-288.
222. York DH, Legan M, Benner S. Watts C. Further studies with a noninvasive method of intracranial pressure estimation. Neurosurg, 1984, 14:456-461.
223. York DH, Pulliam MW, Rosenfeld JG, Watts C. Relationship between visual evoked potentials and intracranial pressure. J Neurosurg, 1981, 55:909-916.
224. Zuccarello M, Fiore DL, Pardatscher K, Martini A, Paolin A, Trincia G, Andrioli GC. Importance of auditory brain stem responses in the CT diagnosis of traumatic brainstem lesions. Am J Neuroradiol, 1983, 4:481-483.

Chapter 7

Post-Traumatic Epilepsy and Medico-Legal Implications of Epileptic, Aggressive, and Criminal States

John R. Hughes

POST-TRAUMATIC EPILEPSY (PTE)

Significant Trauma (Concussion)

Trauma here refers to concussion: a closed head injury of sufficient severity to produce unconsciousness and/or amnesia. Obviously, open head injuries with penetration through the skull will also be included as significant trauma, although consciousness may not be lost in some instances.

Early PTE

PTE can be divided into seizures occurring *early* within one week after the trauma and those appearing *later* beyond that first week [58]. Jennett and Teasdale [60] have reported that 5% of patients with non-missile head injuries admitted to a hospital fall into the early category. Patients with early attacks include some young children, but usually are adults with severe trauma, including those with prolonged post-traumatic amnesia, depressed skull fracture, and/or intracranial hemorrhage. The inclusion of children in this category is indicated by the data of Hendrick and Harris [48] who reported a 7% incidence of early seizures of head-injured victims under age 5,

133

11% of whom were under age 1. The majority (60%) of patients with early epilepsy have their first seizure within 24 hours, and in slightly less than one-half of these, the seizure occurs in the first hour. Most (two-thirds) of the patients will have more than one seizure and one in 10 will actually develop status epilepticus, seen in 20% of children under age 5 who have early attacks. The type of seizure is generalized without a focal component (40%) as often as it is focal motor without generalization (40%). Since early PTE is often associated with *severe* trauma, it may point to intracranial complications like hemorrhage and increase the risk of late epilepsy.

Late PTE

This form of PTE is seen in only 5% of all patients admitted to the hospital after non-missile head injury, similar to the incidence in early PTE [60]. Also, as in the early form, there is a higher risk with intracranial hemorrhage or compound depressed fracture. If only severe injuries are considered, 15% of patients develop seizure in about one year, and nearly 90% have an intracranial hemorrhage or depressed fracture. As time progresses, more patients show their first seizure: 27% will appear within three months of injury, 56% within the first year, 69% the second year, 78% the third, 82% the fourth, 86% the fifth, and 89% by the sixth year.

Phillips [88] reported slightly different values: 55% of those who were going to develop PTE will have manifested a clinical seizure in 3 months, 82% in one year, 85% in two years, 97% in four years, reaching 100% in 11 years. Jasper and Penfield [57] had slightly different statistics, with 46% during the first year, 63% in three years, and 80% within a five year period. The recent data of Weiss et al [126] shows values of 53%, 77%, and 84% for one, three, and five years, with 99% at 15 years.

Perr [86] found the incidence of seizures after head injury varies from 0.1% to 50%, depending on the medico-legal investigation reviewed. Perr also pointed out that "idiopathic" epilepsy is 15 to 20 times more common than post-traumatic seizures. This statistic appears to provide some perspective on the relative incidence of post-traumatic epilepsy. However, careful histories of epileptics seem to reduce the incidence of genuine "idiopathic" epilepsy, which may be less common than once thought. Hyslop [55] studied 715 head injuries introduced for litigation, and the number of frankly fraudulent cases outnumbered the true cases of post-traumatic epilepsy by more than 2 to 1. A reasonable possibility of post-traumatic epilepsy was found in 8.6% of the cases, but only 20% of these could actually be verified.

If early and late PTE are not divided, then 76% have their seizure within the first year [60]. The type of late seizure is clearly focal in 40%, similar in incidence to that seen in early seizures. In 20% of late attacks, the seizures are temporal lobe or complex-partial in type. Absence attacks with bilaterally synchronous spike and wave complexes of the cortico-reticular or generalized type are not encountered as a form of PTE. The latter form has a strong inheritance, especially from the mother, and patients with absence attacks with a history of some type of head injury do not have seizures that can be considered as PTE.

As to persistence of seizures, three-fourths of the patients with PTE will continue to have seizures for years after their onset, especially patients with a temporal lobe or complex-partial type and also those with a delayed onset for more than two years after injury. If the seizures took a relatively long time to develop, probably from a slow insidious glial proliferation, then they usually take a long time to control. In seizure control, the term "remission" is better than "cessation" in these cases, since once seizures occur in a given patient, a relatively low threshold for further attacks may be found. Given a lower threshold to develop PTE in the first place, then possibly even after a seizure-free period, another attack may occur at any time when conditions further lower this threshold.

Jennett and Teasdale [60] have pointed out three factors that significantly increase the risk of late epilepsy: early epilepsy, acute intracranial hematoma, and depressed skull fracture. Long post-traumatic amnesia (> 24 hrs) is not a very significant factor unless it is coupled with early seizures (30% vs 2%). Although early PTE may be slightly more common in children than in adults, children are less affected by early epilepsy as a risk for the later form. In patients with a depressed fracture, Jennett and Teasdale [60] point to four significant features: torn dura, focal clinical signs, long post-traumatic amnesia (> 24 hrs), and early seizures. Factors that seem to be less important are the site of fracture, whether bone fragments are removed or replaced, and elevation of the fracture. Varying combinations of the four risk factors are associated with a very wide range of risks of late epilepsy from 3% (only focal signs) to 70% (torn dura, long amnesia, and early seizures).

The EEG would be expected to play a role in predicting late epilepsy, especially by detecting the development of a discharging focus. Jennett and Teasdale [60] point out that EEG abnormalities usually decrease in time (2 year period) after the injury but do so less in patients who develop late epilepsy. Patients with late PTE had an abnormal EEG at one year (83%) and two years (73%), as opposed to 76% and 46% with no late epilepsy. The authors point out that significant differences between the latter two groups are seen only after one year, thereby rendering the test less useful for early prediction. They also mention other investigators in the literature who consider EEG not particularly helpful in predicting late epilepsy [20,116,123]. One major point must be made in defense of the EEG: it is only the sharp wave or spike focus that relates directly to seizures, and this latter type of abnormal activity usually requires a sleep record for its appearance. In most of the studies mentioned, sleep records were not performed on all or even most patients; without such records, no valid comment can be made whether a discharging focus exists or not.

PTE in the Military

Overview

Military data is important in studying PTE because of the large number of open head injuries with penetrating missiles and dural tears that have been studied. Table

7.1 shows the incidence of seizures from World War I [3,26], World War II [88,99, 121,130], Korea [15,125], and the Vietnam conflict [17], totalling more than 7000 casualties. This table demonstrates that roughly one-third of head-injured soldiers have developed PTE, regardless of the war and the date. Table 7.1 also shows that dural penetration is an important variable: the mean seizure incidence is 43% with and 14% without such a penetration. A recent report by Weiss et al [126] shows that this value increases to 50% when the soldiers (520) with penetrating injuries are followed for 15 years. The 1030 (Vietnam) American patients studied by Cavenass et al [17] had a mean age of 21.3 years at injury, resulting from missile fragments (75%), gunshot wounds (16%), vehicular accidents (4%), and others (3%). Further characteristics of these injuries (with or without PTE) include the absence of unconsciousness in 55%, light comatose state but with response to command in 20%, and a deeper comatose state with response only to pain in 25%. The head injuries were only fractures in 17%, penetration into a single lobe of the brain in 42%, and into multiple lobes in 41%.

Details of the Head Injury

One important variable is the *extent and degree of brain damage* to determine the probability of PTE. Of the 172 patients with only a skull fracture, 22% developed seizures, less than the 28% (of 437) who had some penetration into a *single* lobe [17]. The greatest incidence at 44% was with penetration into multiple lobes, which increased to 59% when the penetration was completely through the different lobes. If only the early seizures during the first week are considered, then no significant differences were noted with regard to extent of injury since 5% of the fractures, 3% of the single lobe penetrations, and 6% of the multiple lobe injuries developed early seizures. For later seizures, Aird et al [1] have indicated a 2% incidence with concussion, 7% with contusion or hemorrhage, 12% with coma > 24 hours, and 40% to 50% with an open injury. Other data [16] demonstrates the general point that an increased incidence of seizure is associated with an increasing amount of brain damage. Strong association includes 7% with seizures after a head injury without neurological deficit, 10% if loss of consciousness occurred for 1 to 6 hours, 20% after a dural penetration but no unconsciousness, 39% after focal damage but no dural tear, 51% after focal damage with a dural tear, and, finally, 57% after severe focal damage and also a dural penetration.

Loss of consciousness (LOC) has proven to be one of the most reliable indices of brain damage according to Caveness et al [17]. This is especially so if a long LOC was documented with focal damage, accompanied by an increased seizure incidence [16]. Among patients maintaining alertness, 28% developed seizures, lower than the 38% in those responding only to commands, which was lower than the 42% if the responses were only to painful stimuli [17]. These latter values show a statistically significant difference ($p < 0.001$). In the case of early seizures within the first week, significant differences ($p = 0.01$) were also found, as attacks developed in 2.8% of

Table 7.1. Incidence of Seizures in Military Head Injury

War	Nationality	No.	%		Dural tear		No tear
WWI	German	1990	38%	(5 yr)	50%		19%
	English	317			45%		23%
WWII	English	2820	–		45%	(5 yr)	6%
	American	739	28%		36%		14%
Korea	American	407	24%	(5 yr)	40%)		16%
			31%	(10yr)	(50%)		(20%)
Vietnam	American	1030	33%		36%		22%
Totals		7303	33.7%		43.1%		13.9%

those alert contrasted with the 4.8% who responded to commands and 7.5% who responded only to pain.

The *location of the brain damage* was another important variable in the Vietnam data, but not in the Jennett and Teasdale data. The closer the lesion was to the central sulcus, the greater was the possibility of seizures developing from the damage. If hemorrhage or CNS infection occurred, these factors increased the probability of seizures [17].

Details of the Seizure

The *latency of onset* of PTE shows a steep curve for the first year and a decreased slope after the second year. The monthly rate of new seizure cases (344) as a percentage of head-injured (1030) victims in the Vietnam conflict and also the new cases (109) from the Korean campaign (356) indicate that 7% to 9% of injured personnel had their first seizure within the first month, 2% to 3% in the next 6 months, and 1% or less thereafter. The early seizures within the first week seemed less related to the details of the injury than the seizures occurring after the first week. The recent report of Weiss et al [126] indicates three groups in terms of seizure onset: the first group (4%) developed attacks within a month, the largest group (76%) with a mean latency of 11 months, and 20% with a mean of 7.7 years.

The *frequency of seizures* in the roughly one-third of the head injured who developed attacks divided into thirds. Over the 10 years of follow-up of 109 cases with seizures (Korea), one-third had only a few (1 to 3 attacks), one-third had a moderate number (4 to 30), and one-third had many (> 30). One important point is that once established, the frequency of seizures seemed not to change and remained relatively constant.

The *duration* of the seizure disorder is reflected in the data showing the aforementioned steep curve for onset of new seizures compared to the less steep curve for the cessation of previous attacks. After 5 years, these two curves were parallel. The difference between the two curves of onset and cessation represented those still having attacks. At the 10 year follow-up, one half of those who had seizures in the past had stopped their attacks.

The *relationship between latency, frequency, and duration* of seizures was then investigated. One important point was that a greater frequency of seizure was related to a greater persistency. This point fits a useful generalization in epileptology, viz., seizures beget seizures. If only very few attacks had occurred, then further seizures were less likely. The relationship between latency of onset and persistency was interesting, especially because of a common view that seizures occurring soon after head injury tend not to persist [3]. In the series of Jennett [59], 25% to 35% of the early seizures persisted into later attacks, and in the series of Caveness [16], a similar 31% of the early attacks persisted to the fourth year. This was later reported as slightly over 50% in the Vietnam material [17]. However, a higher incidence (68%) was found if the seizures began after the first week. Thus, it is a matter of relative degree as to the extent to which seizures persist, relative to their time of onset after head injury.

The seizure pattern was then reviewed and focal seizures were found to be the most common, tending to occur more than those that were always generalized. In particular, one quarter of the seizures were focal from the onset; one half were focal at first, later showing secondary generalization; and only one quarter were always generalized [17]. No bilaterally synchronous spike and wave complex of the cortico-reticular or generalized type (absence seizures) were found by Caveness in either the Korean or Vietnam series.

Details of the Individual

Correlations can be found between extent of brain damage and incidence of seizure, but clearly some cases with relatively minor head trauma develop seizures and some with major damage do not ever develop attacks. Also, once attacks occur and their frequency is apparent, there is a tendency for that same frequency to persist for a given individual regardless of the anticonvulsant medication given. In addition, the cessation of attacks did not seem related to the degree of damage nor to the latency. These facts lead to the conclusion that there must be something intrinsic about the individual which helps determine the reactivity of the brain to the head injury in the form of seizures. That characteristic can be referred to as a multifactorial genetic trait or an inherited threshold to seizure. This factor probably explains why one third of military head injury victims developed seizures in each of the periods — World War I, World War II, Korea, Vietnam — even with improved handling of wounds and anticonvulsant medication. If this genetic trait plays a major role, then the military and civilian experiences might prove to be somewhat similar, even though the military data often includes more severe injuries, especially more dural penetrations.

For early seizure (< 1 wk), the Vietnam experience (1030 head injuries) was 4.4%, compared to 4.6% of the 1000 patients with mild injuries in the Oxford civilian series [59]. Excluding these early cases, the cumulative incidence of seizure patients within

5 years was 27.9% from Vietnam [17], comparable to the similar 28.6% incidence from 2005 depressed skull fractures of Glasgow and 420 hematomas from Rotterdam [50].

The development of seizures each year over the 5 years shows the cumulative percentages to be 67%, 89%, 95%, 98%, 100% from the Vietnam casualties of Caveness, quite similar to the 66%, 81%, 91%, 96%, and 100% from the Glasgow cases of Jennett. Thus, the data suggests that a certain pool of individuals exists with a relatively low threshold to seizure, and after some significant head injury, these same patients tend to develop seizure, regardless of any particular circumstances. This report has emphasized that certain conditions or factors tend to elicit seizures more than others. Additional data argues for a core of patients who show evidence of a low threshold toward seizures, regardless of specific environmental factors.

Prevention of Seizures

Surgery
Surgery is usually undertaken in patients with open injuries. Decompression is done for debridement, dural closure, minimization of sinus penetration, cerebral edema, and infection. Although epileptogenic foci can be removed in some patients with significant success usually after a period of time, the military experience has usually been that this approach is not very practical in the acute or subacute phase.

Prophylactic anticonvulsant medication
The usefulness of anticonvulsants to *prevent the development* of seizures following head injuries has been controversial. The Vietnam experience reported by Caveness et al [17] was disappointing. In 524 patients, the medication was interrupted and in another 335, these drugs were continuously given each day and monitored for more than one year. Nevertheless, seizure incidence was not significantly different between these two groups. This was the case if all seizure patients were considered (49% vs 52%), only late seizure patients (51% vs 49%), or all head injuries (20% vs 30%). In 84%, the drugs were given IM in the first 24 hours (phenytoin 300 to 400 mg/day in 75%, phenytoin and 96 mg/day of phenobarbital in 20%, or phenobarbital alone in 3%). The possibility that IV administration was necessary to obtain quicker therapeutic levels was considered in this study. However, the majority of seizures began beyond the time when IV administration should have played any significant role. A more recent report of Weiss et al [126] also showed that phenytoin for at least a year after a penetrating injury had no overall decrease in the ultimate seizure incidence, although possibly it delayed the onset.

The past history of efforts to protect the head-injured from later seizures by prophylactic anticonvulsant drugs is full of conflicting results. On the one hand, Birkmayer [8] reported that among 150 patients, phenytoin (200 mg/day) after 7 years led to only a 6% seizure incidence, in contrast to 51% among the unmedicated controls. On the other hand, Rish and Caveness [96] reported that for early seizures the 1.6% incidence with phenytoin (300 to 400 mg) and phenobarbital (100 mg) was not significantly different (p = 0.07) from the 3.7% who were untreated. These authors actually concluded that "prophylaxis against early post-traumatic fits may not be practical or desirable." Popek [93] and Servit [102] reported that a 2.1% seizure incidence among 143 with phenytoin (160 to 240 mg) and phenobarbital (30 to 60 mg) contrasted with the 25% in the controls. The follow-up period was 3 years, even to 10 years in 37% of those followed, when significant differences continued to be seen. Penry [87], however, could not confirm the results. Wohms and Wyler [134] studied 50 patients on phenytoin (400 mg) and 10% developed seizures, in contrast to the 50% incidence of 12 control patients. Blackwood et al [9] dealt with a similar population with severe head injuries and split 165 of these cases into the phenytoin group (84) or placebo group (81). Both groups had four patients develop seizures during the first year and both had two more in the second year. Although EEGs were done on only a minority of the patients, they were not helpful in predicting the patients who would develop clinical attacks.

Similar patients with severe head injury had been studied by Young et al [136] who used phenytoin IV (11 mg/kg) at first, then IM (13 mg/kg), and later oral (8.8 mg/kg), trying to obtain therapeutic levels as quickly as possible. Since only 6% of these patients developed seizures during the first year and the literature would have predicted approximately a 25% incidence among untreated controls, the study was judged as indicating a prophylactic effect. However, the need for a prospective double blind study was seen. A double blind study was published [137], in which 244 severely injured patients were given either phenytoin (IV, IM, oral) or a placebo. The drug and placebo groups both showed a 3.7% incidence of seizures from 5 of 136 in the drug group and 4 of 108 in the placebo group. Other authors, like Johnson et al [61] and Bouzarth and Goldman [11] have criticized these negative conclusions — mainly on statistical grounds, with such small numbers of patients involved (5 and 4), but also that some patients did not have therapeutic blood levels when their seizures occurred. Thus, the epileptologist is left with conflicting data regarding the efficacy of prophylactic anticonvulsant medication on the severely head-injured victim.

This reviewer would encourage trials with carbamazepine (Tegretol), an excellent anticonvulsant with a short half-life that can build up to therapeutic levels in a short period of time. Three-quarters of these head-injured patients had seizures which began as focal attacks; carbamazepine should be considered because its greatest efficacy is for the focal or partial seizure, mainly from the temporal lobe. The usefulness of phenytoin and phenobarbital must also be considered and they should not be abandoned as some data has demonstrated their effectiveness in preventing PTE.

The final question may be the designation of those patients who should be given these medications. Like all similar questions, the risk-benefit ratio must be considered. The drugs that have been suggested are safe in the great majority of patients and the side effects are usually minimal. Since the benefit of these drugs has been shown by a number of studies, then the safest suggestion is to use these medications, especially in the severely injured patients at risk. Finally, it is important to spell out the kind of patient who should be given these drugs. Servit [102], Young et al [136], and Caveness [16] all recommend them for the patient with focal neurological signs or dural penetration or long coma (Servit: > 3 hours, Young: > 24 hours). With coma greater than 24 hours and dural tear, 40% develop seizures. This data argues strongly for a concerted attempt to use prophylactic anticonvulsants in these patients to prevent later PTE. Other factors which are added to the list are the aforementioned early seizures [16,136] or hemorrhage or depressed fracture [137]. Three other factors are added by Servit as an attempt to stress early or genetic predisposition: abnormal birth, family history of seizures, and febrile seizures. Weiss et al [126] have shown the following factors to increase the probability of seizures: unconsciousness with injury, retained metal fragments, hematoma, initial hemiparesis, aphasia, and lesions in the right vertex cortex, right corona radiata, frontal white matter, left convexity, and left temporal white matter. The reviewer would add the presence on EEG of clear, paroxysmal discharges as another guide. This is because a discharging focus is probably required for these seizures to develop, and past studies have not thoroughly examined this variable. The final conclusion is that the usefulness of prophylactic anticonvulsant medication should be encouraged, if any one of the above factors is found in the history of a head-injured victim, in hopes of preventing post-traumatic epilepsy.

MEDICO-LEGAL ASPECTS OF HEAD INJURY

Electroencephalography is a fine objective tool to confirm PTE and also a very useful tool to determine the extent of brain damage after any head injury. We live in a world of litigation and all electroencephalographers must be prepared to testify in a court of law regarding EEGs they have interpreted. There are many ways in which we may find ourselves in court to testify as an expert witness; among them are cases of head injury with or without possible post-traumatic epilepsy and also examples of a seizure disorder as a possible contributing factor in a given crime of violence. Furthermore, an electroencephalographer may be called upon to provide evidence regarding the possible incompetency or legal insanity of a patient.

Difference Between Mental Incompetency and Insanity

In his outline on the differences between legal insanity and criminal incompetency, Morse [82] points out that insanity represents a more drastic, severe, and more general condition than criminal incompetency — which relates to a specific condition. The term *insanity* is associated with the time of *commission* of the crime, whereas the term *mental incompetency* refers to the accused's behavior before and during the trial and after a judgment has been entered, but before the pronouncement of a sentence.

Tests for incompetency refer to an inability on the part of the individual charged with an offense (1) to understand the nature and purpose of the proceedings against him, (2) to assist in his defense, and (3) to understand the nature and purpose of any sentence that may be imposed on him by a court of law. As a legal term, insanity refers to inability on the part of the individual charged with a crime to understand the difference between right and wrong. A defendant declared insane is one who is judged to have been incapable of avoiding the act in question because of the absence of "free will" at the time of the crime. This definition thus implies that the crime was associated with some type of mental disorder. Electroencephalographers may find it difficult to provide testimony providing evidence on these two legal conditions, but one may be called upon to present data that could have some bearing on either condition.

The Insanity Defense

McNaghten Rule

In 1843, Daniel McNaghten attempted to assassinate Sir Robert Peel, the Prime Minister of England. The response of Lord Chief Justice Findal in *Rex vs McNaghten* [a] had been for years the model for an insanity defense in the U.S. and had stated, "To establish a defense on the grounds of insanity, it must be clearly proved that, at the time of the committing of the act, the party accused was labouring under such a defect of reason from a disorder of the mind, as not to know the nature and quality of the act he was doing; or if he did know it, that he did not know he was doing what was wrong." This "McNaghten Rule" served for almost a century, but the criticism was that mentally ill individuals can sometimes distinguish between right and wrong, but may not be able to control their wrongful actions. Thus, some states supplemented the "right from wrong" test with the "irresistible impulse" standard.

Durham Rule

In 1954, Judge Bazelon of the U.S. Court of Appeals for the District of Columbia rejected the McNaghten rule as too narrow, requesting a broader test which provided that "an accused is not criminally responsible if his unlawful act was the product of a mental disease or defect." This is now known as the Durham Rule. This new rule was too general and broad and was an insufficient guide to juries, according to Hagan [45], while the McNaghten rule was too narrow. Thus a new standard arose in the 1960s.

American Law Institute Standard

This standard states that "a person is not responsible for criminal conduct if at the time of such conduct as a result of mental disease or defect he lacks substantial capacity either to appreciate the criminality of his conduct or to conform his conduct to the requirements of the law." The standard absolved from criminal punishment those mentally ill individuals who understood what they did yet were driven to crime by delusions, fears, or compulsions. This standard is now used in the majority of states, according to Hagan [45].

Guilty but Mentally Ill

In 1975, Michigan was the first to replace "not guilty by reason of insanity" by "guilty but mentally ill." In 1981, Indiana and Illinois adopted the latter standard, and the next year Alaska, Delaware, Georgia, Kentucky, and New Mexico passed similar legislation.

Abolition of Insanity Defense

In Montana, the insanity defense was considered admissible only when relevant to prove "a defendant did not have the state of mind which was an element of that offense." This refers to a mental state which would not be consistent with the crime, exemplified by a murderer who had no malice at all toward the victim and viewed the victim as only an object. This standard is similar to the Federal approach in the form of the proposed Violent Crimes Enforcement Act of 1982 which states "It is a defense to a prosecution under any Federal Statute that the defendant, as a result of mental disease or defect, lacked the state of mind required as an element of the offense charge. Mental disease or defect does not otherwise constitute a defense." Thus, only under very specific conditions is insanity a defense according to this proposal.

The EEG as Legal Evidence

When electroencephalographers testify in court, they will probably be asked to define the term *electroencephalogram*. Some states include within their legal statutes such a definition. In 1953, the Court of Appeals of the State of Louisiana, for example, in *Betz vs Travis Insurance Company* [b] defined EEG as a "graphic recording of the electrical currents developed in the cortex by brain action and by this examination it can be determined whether [a person] actually suffered any damage to his brain."

There is usually no difficulty in introducing the EEG as legal evidence, and a higher court in the State of Illinois ruled that EEG can thus be presented as evidence. This particular case was *Melford vs Gaus and Brown Construction Company* [c] in 1958 from an Appellate Court. Also, during the next year there were other Annotations [d] regarding the admissibility of an EEG as evidence. In Federal courts and in states having legislation similar to the Uniform Business Records as Evidence Act, it has been held that such statutes authorize the introduction of EEG records because they do qualify as business records, as exemplified in *Croll vs John Hancock Mutual Life*

Insurance Company, 1952 [e], *Kramer vs John Hancock Mutual Life Insurance Company*, 1957 [f], and *Young vs Liddington*, 1957 [g].

At least one high court has decided that it is prejudicial to exclude EEGs when they are relevant, as noted in *Maypole vs B. Crystal and Son Inc.*, 1943 [h]. In this instance the Appellate Division of the Supreme Court in New York held that the EEG tracings and the interpretation thereof by a medical expert were admissible as evidence, and the court claimed: "the [lower] court committed error in excluding the testimony of plaintiff's medical witness as to the condition or conditions for which the electroencephalogram was a test. It was also error to exclude the electroencephalogram and the records respecting it made in the regular course of business." In the Betz suit [b] previously mentioned, the Louisiana Court of Appeals reversed the judgment of the lower court and remanded the case (sent the case back to the lower court) to permit the introduction of further evidence in the form of the EEG tracings.

Woolsey and Goldner [135] have made some suggestions to electroencephalographers to ensure proper identification of an EEG record introduced into court. For example, they suggest that the EEG must be marked at the time it is taken with the name and address of the patient, the place of the test, and the name of the technician. They point out that many courts will permit the introduction of the EEG through the testimony of the physician interpreting the record and that the technician need not be present at the trial. On the other hand, a few courts have required the testimony of the technician performing the examination, as in *Quadlander vs Kansas City Public Service Company* [i] and *Hinrichs vs Young* [j]. However, the particular annoying issue of the need for the technician to testify can usually be resolved easily during a pretrial conference.

Gibbs and Gibbs [34] have also made some excellent suggestions for electroencephalographers about to set foot in court. For example, they suggest that a recording that is *likely* to end up in a courtroom should not be cut down for storage. The tracing should be continuous and, if possible, contained within a single pack of paper. They also suggest that the patient or guardian should sign the EEG on the face of the recording as soon as it is completed and in the presence of the technician. If a new pack of paper should be inserted into the EEG during the recording, this second pack should be numbered and identified and also signed by the patient and his/her guardian. The technician should, of course, sign the recording in the presence of the patient or guardian. All signatures should appear on the face of the recording together with the data and all pertinent information related to the recording.

On the question of the need for the electroencephalographer to be present at the time the EEG was taken, the 1961 case of *Frey vs State* [k] decided by the Court of Appeals of the State of Texas is relevant. A Dr. Crowley testified that the EEG tracings from a given defendant were normal, but a complaint was registered in court that Crowley's interpretation could have been in error because he was not present during the recording of the electroencephalogram. However, Dr. Crowley testified that he was in charge of the EEG laboratory, the EEG machine was in good working condition, and the tracing was taken by a technician under his supervision. The court concluded that no error was shown in this instance. Each electroencephalographer should be prepared to be challenged on the point of his absence during the actual recording, but the simple statement will usually suffice that the physician is generally not present for any of these recordings, which are taken by technicians under supervision of the electroencephalographer.

EEG in Head Injury in Medical Legal Issues

The most typical example of an instance in which the electroencephalographer will be called to testify in court is on the question of a significant head injury, usually defined as a blow sufficient to cause unconsciousness (concussion). Mark and Ervin [74] have stated that even as far back as 1968, there were approximately 3 million motor vehicle accidents, and head injury was the most frequent lethal injury in such accidents. This one fact should give the reader a clear impression of the magnitude of the problem of head injury in the United States.

One of the major problems in assessing the significance of any abnormal EEG pattern in a patient who has suffered a head injury is that very rarely do electroencephalographers have evidence of the status of the EEG prior to the head injury. This point is obviously important in order to assess the significance of any EEG abnormality, and it may become even more crucial in a court of law. Therefore, since rarely do we have the EEG before the accident in any given patient, the electroencephalographer must use statistical probabilities, based on previous evidence and experience, to judge the likelihood that any given abnormality may be the result of a head injury, as opposed to its presence before the injury. Gibbs and his colleagues as early as 1944 [36] provided some statistics that could be of value in this instance. For example, the general conclusion was drawn that a focal EEG abnormality in patients with head trauma strongly suggested the presence of "brain damage;" more specifically, if a *generalized* abnormality was present three months or more after a *mild* head injury, the changes were 6 to 1 that the abnormality antedated the head injury. Further statistics in this study revealed that if a *normal* EEG existed three months or later after the head injury, the chances were 53 to 8 that the patient did *not* have post-traumatic epilepsy. Gibbs and his colleagues also indicated that if the EEG were normal, the brain could still be damaged, and the statistics were that only 3 in 60 patients fell into this category. Finally, if a *paroxysmal* abnormality was noted more than three months after a head injury, the chances were 27 to 2 that the patient had some type of epileptic condition. If the patient had clinical seizures and also a focal paroxysmal abnormality more than three months after a head injury, the chances were 21 to 7 that seizures were the result of the trauma, rather than the result of some other factor [36]. These probabilities, of course, are based on statistics of that particular study, and such statistics are useful in making intelligent judgments and predictions. This data was reported over 45 years ago and needs to be updated.

Courjon [22] has summarized the same kinds of probabilities (but less specific) based on more recent evidence. His general conclusion was that if an EEG is normal or shows only a very mild abnormality immediately after a head injury and continues to show a normal tracing, an organic lesion is very unlikely but still is possible. On the other hand, long-lasting EEG abnormalities with slow abatement are characteristic of major organic cerebral injuries. The secondary deterioration of an EEG suggests post-traumatic complications such as subdural hematoma, abscess, or seizures, or could also suggest non-traumatic disease. In these instances, complementary clinical investigations are, of course, definitely required. Persistent EEG abnormalities without any abatement suggest the same two possibilities, namely: post-traumatic complications or non-traumatic disease.

If an EEG is performed *early* in the post-traumatic stage, there are usually good correlations between the clinical signs and the EEG abnormality [62]. If the EEG is done only *late* in the post-traumatic stage, the electroencephalographer is often asked to state the degree of probability that the head injury was the cause of the abnormality. This decision is more difficult. However, one can help to determine the extent of abnormality, to localize the lesion, and to predict the possibility of late post-traumatic complications [38]. As Courjon [22] points out, one cannot verify subjective symptoms such as headaches, dizziness, and post-traumatic psychiatric disturbances by an abnormal EEG, nor is it possible from a normal tracing to disprove the presence of those same symptoms. On the other hand, a normal EEG in the face of clear neurological deficits suggests that further clinical recovery is not expected. A normal EEG during waking and *sleep* cannot, of course, guarantee that seizures will not occur [20,76], but it offers some evidence against this possibility. If the EEG is abnormal, this finding may be a clue for the development of late complications, especially seizures.

A spike or sharp-wave focus at the site of the original traumatic lesion usually is associated with late epilepsy. But there are some patients who never do develop clinical seizures even with a persistent irritative EEG pattern in the form of a spike or sharp-wave focus. If clear seizures do exist, the EEG can assist in determining the cause [33]. Courjon [22] has summarized that in head-injured patients with seizures, a slow-wave focus, without any generalized abnormality, provides strong evidence for post-traumatic seizures, but a normal EEG may also (rarely) occur under the same circumstances. According to Courjon, frequent spikes, in addition to a severe generalized abnormality, suggest a non-traumatic origin for a seizure disorder. Also, bilaterally synchronous 3/sec spike and wave complexes are not compatible with post-traumatic epilepsy [92].

Courjon has pointed out that two EEG patterns are occasionally suspected of being a post-traumatic pattern: (1) low-voltage records and (2) posterior theta rhythms. However, Meyer-Mickeleit [78] found low-voltage EEGs in the normal population as often as in chronic head injuries and found that such low-voltage records were often the result of anxiety, tension, or expectancy of the patient. Vogel [120] found that low-voltage records usually could be considered an inherited variant of cerebral activity, as was also the case for posterior theta activity. Other studies would argue strongly that low-voltage patterns and posterior theta activity cannot necessarily be attributed to head injury [100].

EEG Abnormality in Criminals

A number of studies have been performed on criminals to determine if these individuals have an increased incidence of abnormal EEG patterns. Variability seems to characterize most of the studies. Silverman [105] found that prisoners showed a 53% incidence of EEG abnormality, but Gibbs et al [35] investigated a larger group of prisoners and found no significant abnormalities. Kennard et al [63] reported a greater incidence of abnormal EEGs in "criminal psychopaths" than in controls, and they emphasized excessive theta activity. Hill and Pond [53] indicated that slightly more than one-half of accused murderers had an abnormal EEG, and Hill [52] published a more specific report on 110 murderers, claiming excessive theta activity in 22% and posterior temporal slow wave activity in 8%. These percentages were greater than found in controls, but there was no increased incidence of spikes in the prisoners.

Some authors have reported a relatively low incidence of EEG abnormality among prisoners. One example is the report of Winkler and Kove [132] on 55 prisoners with a homicidal history in which only 24% were said to have an abnormal record. Likewise Levy and Kennard [69] reported only a 15% incidence of abnormal EEGs among both violent and nonviolent murderers. Small [108] reported on 100 individuals who had committed felonies and found an EEG abnormality in 33%; however, 77% had some type of organic dysfunction, either in the form of seizure history, head injury, neurological signs, or an abnormal psychological examination. She concluded that a single EEG alone could easily be misleading.

A very high incidence of EEG abnormality has also been reported among criminals. For example, Stafford-Clark and Taylor [110] reported on 64 murderers and found that 73% of them showed an abnormal EEG, especially in motiveless crimes. This value contrasted with a 25% incidence of abnormality among the controls in prison [111]. In that latter study, an 83% incidence of abnormal EEGs was found in aggressive psychopaths in prison. Among 411 prisoners, Silverman [105] reported a 75% incidence of EEG abnormality, especially among those who had committed psychopathic crimes. Williams [131] reported a study of prisoners with repetitive assaultive behavior and found that they had a significantly higher incidence of abnormal EEGs than those whose crime was only a single act. Similarly, Levy [68] found the incidence of EEG abnormality in recidivists to be twice as high as in persons who were imprisoned for the first time.

Alström [2] reported on 345 male epileptics and compared that group to 42,000 males in the general population with regard to the incidence of these two groups in the penal register. The register included 7.0% of the epileptics and also 4.8% of males in the general population, suggesting that epileptics may more frequently find themselves behind bars. Violent crimes were committed in 17% of those who were epileptic compared to 11% in the general population. Alström was careful to point out that no crimes were committed during a seizure. In 1978, Riley and Niedermeyer [95] studied 229 EEGs of 212 violent patients, but only 6.6% showed mild abnormalities without any demonstrating epileptiform patterns. The conclusion from these authors was that there was no EEG evidence for an increased incidence of epilepsy in a non-incarcerated group of patients who were referred specifically for outbursts of violent and antisocial behavior.

Some studies suggest that the incidence of EEG abnormality may vary according to the nature of the crime. In the study by Stafford-Clark and Taylor [110], those who had committed motivated murder under considerable provocation had a 17% incidence of abnormal EEGs, similar to that in the general population, and those who had murdered accidentally while committing some other felony showed a slightly higher (25%) incidence. These values contrast with explosive psychopaths who committed murder without motive and 73% of these criminals showed abnormal EEGs. The highest incidence was 86%, found among those who were obviously insane at the time they committed their crimes. These studies suggest that a higher incidence of EEG abnormality is related to an increasing degree of violent (perhaps insane) behavior. In a study conducted by Walton [123] on the EEGs of 20 murderers, 35% were found abnormal. Although this incidence was lower than in most other studies, it was higher than those committing other kinds of crimes or in the general population.

As Curran [24] has emphasized, the possession of an abnormal EEG might thus become a criminal asset, and it is important for all electroencephalographers to keep this point in mind. If an EEG is abnormal, this fact, of course, does not constitute any proof at all of the existence of epilepsy as an extenuating factor in a crime, as was pointed out in the 1961 case of *Armstead vs State of Maryland* [1]. In this court case, a medical expert testified that certain abnormal EEG findings did not establish a lack of criminal responsibility. The conviction was confirmed largely on the strength of this expert testimony.

The possibility that abnormal EEGs may be prevalent in criminals introduces the idea that violent behavior could be the result of some type of brain damage. However, this is not to suggest that all violence is caused by individuals with damaged brains. Mark and Ervin [74] emphasize that there is a kind of violent behavior related to brain malfunction which probably has its origins in the environment, "but once the brain structures have been permanently affected," the violent behavior can no longer be modified by manipulating psychological or social influences. Mark and Ervin also pointed out that experiments have indicated a definable neural system which organizes affective and directive attack behavior and that this system is linked to the limbic brain. They further point out that man frequently has aggressive actions which are not really the result of a simple instinct but constitute one of the many different varieties of behavior characteristic of Homo sapiens. If the brain of man is organically damaged, then the capacity for violence is said to exceed that of any other animal.

Mark and Ervin [74] claim that chromosomal studies help to provide evidence that organicity may be involved with such violent behavior. For example, those with XXY chromosomes frequently show behavioral disorders and those with an XYY chromosomal pattern more frequently show antisocial behavior. According to the review of Mark and Ervin, the XY siblings of those with an XYY pattern usually do not have a record of breaking the law, but the siblings of the XY inmates are frequently in jail. These findings suggest that the *environment* of the inmates with the XY chromosomal pattern plays a very important role, while it is the specific abnormal *chromosomal pattern* in the XYY individuals that seems related to their antisocial behavior. The relationship between antisocial behavior and the XYY pattern has more recently been challenged as a statistical artifact [91] or as a problem related to decreased intelligence [133].

Epilepsy in Criminals

Gunn and his colleagues [41] have carried out studies for decades on the prevalence of epilepsy in British prisoners and in 1977 provided details in a monograph, summarized in Table 7.2. Although the prevalence of epilepsy in the general population has also been a matter of significant controversy and values do vary in this table, Gunn concluded that the prevalence of epilepsy in imprisoned males was approximately three times higher than in the general population. Earlier in 1971, Gunn and Bonn [42] had sampled 5000 males incarcerated in England and Wales and found the prevalence rate for seizures as 8.8/1000, similar to some of the values listed in Table 7.2. Of the epileptics, 17% had committed acts of violence, compared to 11% of the non-epileptics who had also committed acts of violence. However, the latter difference was not statistically significant. The same two investigators carried out another survey in order to judge the prevalence of epilepsy among inmates at one given time and found 8.7/1000 among nearly 31,000 prisoners. This prevalence rate was nearly two times the rate of 4.5/1000 reported for the general population in a 1960 survey by the College of General Practitioners. One of the many problems in these studies was to define epilepsy so specifically that prisoners would not be included just because they attended a seizure clinic, had EEGs performed, or had been treated with anticonvulsants. With a more operational and strict definition of epilepsy, Gunn and Fenton [43] resurveyed the prisoners and confirmed that 82% of those first considered as having epilepsy probably did have the disorder. The original prevalence value then dropped to 7.2/1000 rather than 8.7, but the value was still nearly double the prevalence rate in the general population.

John R. Hughes

Table 7.2. Epilepsy among Criminals

	Sample Size	Rate/1000 Overall	Rate/1000 15-20 yrs	Rate/1000 Violent Offenders
East (1927)	4000	9 (borstal boys	12 − 4	23
Healy (1929)	1000		67 (recidivists)	
Burt (1944)	200		40 (delinquennts)	
Matheson & Hill (1943)	23925	11 − 6 4 − 1 (females)		
Hill & Pond (1952)	110			160 (murderers)
O'Connell (1960)	50			100 (murderers)
Gibbens & Prince (1962)	532	5 − 6 (female shoplifters)		
West (1963)	100	10 (recidivists)		
Morris & Blom-Cooper (1964)	764			10 (murderers)
Bluglass (1966)	300	10 (prisoners)		
Cowie et al (1968)	328		18 − 9 (girls)	

These figures refer to males except where indicated. (after Gunn 1977)

King and Young [66] determined their prevalence rates in over 1200 inmates of Illinois institutions, based on prescription rates, and they calculated a 1.9% rate, more than three times that in the general population as reported by Hauser and Kurland [46] in a Minnesota city population. This value was similar to the 1.8% rate found by Novick et al [83] among the 1420 prisoners entering the New York City correctional facilities.

These higher prevalence values among prisoners with epilepsy compared to the general population could reflect the higher prevalence of seizures in a deprived urban population, as suggested by the relatively high 1.9% value for epilepsy in black children in an inner city population [103]. As one way to determine the degree of relationship between epilepsy and violent crime, Gunn and Fenton [43] also examined the degree of violence among epileptics compared to a control group and found no significant differences.

As one other way to investigate the relationships between violence and epilepsy, the incidence of "psychomotor" seizures has been studied in delinquent children. Pincus et al [89] studied males who were incarcerated and found 74% of those considered violent had subjective symptoms, suggesting complex partial seizures to the authors, while only 22% of the non-violent males had similar symptoms. On the basis of objective and subjective symptoms, Pincus and his colleagues concluded that slightly over one-half of the violent males had a good chance of having seizures compared to none of the non-violent males. Another study from the same group [70] involved a retrospective chart review of children in juvenile court. Signs or symptoms suggestive of psychomotor epilepsy were reported in 6%, and nearly one-half (44%) of those involved an attack against a person. In a prospective study [71], 78% of incarcerated delinquent boys had one or more signs or symptoms considered by the authors as psychomotor. A significant positive correlation was reported between these signs and symptoms and the degree of violence as judged on a 5-point scale. Two clinicians judged that 11 boys had had a definite and seven a probable psychomotor seizure, the majority of whom had histories of severe CNS trauma or perinatal disorders. Five were thought to have committed violent acts during a seizure and all five were considered violent when seizures were not occurring. Obviously, one problem in these conclusions is the extent to which "psychomotor symptoms" provide sufficient evidence to make a diagnosis of a complex partial seizure. As Stevens [112] has pointed out, the symptoms of schizophrenia, severe disturbances of mood and behavior, and manic-depressive states may manifest clinical characteristics resembling the auras and automatisms of partial complex epilepsy.

Those who are incarcerated tend to come from the underprivileged portions of our society, and it is important to determine the prevalence of epilepsy among them to assess the high incidence of seizures among criminals. Since King and Young [66] had found a 1.9% prevalence of epilepsy among prisoners, Whitman et al [128] inferred that this higher rate is characteristic of the lower socio-economic classes. Many different population surveys in rural Alabama [54], rural Appalachia [6], Iceland [39], Colombia [37], Chile [18], and England [13] would also support this inference. Thus, the relationship between socio-economic status and epilepsy may well explain the higher incidence of epilepsy among prisoners. In other words, lower socio-economic groups demonstrate a relatively high incidence of both epilepsy and also of violent crimes, but there may be no causal relationship between these two phenomena.

Violence in the Interictal State

The relationship between violence and epilepsy can be investigated either by determining the prevalence of violence among epileptics or the prevalence of epilepsy among violent individuals. The former relationship was investigated by Ounsted [85] who studied 100 children with temporal lobe epilepsy, 36% of whom had "outbursts of catastrophic rage." These children also tended to have refractory seizures and many (35%) had a history of severe brain trauma or long-lasting febrile seizures. Children with "pure temporal lobe epilepsy" did not show the rage attacks. Several additional studies suggest that violence was not simply related to epilepsy, but tended to occur with epilepsy only when the seizures began in childhood or adolescence, mainly in institutionalized males with low intelligence level [56,101]. Rodin [97] found 34 (4.8%) "destructive assaultive" patients among 700 at the Lafayette Clinic and Epilepsy Center in Michigan. Destructive assaultive epileptics tended to have more behavioral psychiatric problems with poorer employment records and more evidence of organic cerebral disease than other epileptic patients. Since complex partial seizures were found in only a small minority of the aggressive group, a direct relationship between seizure type and violence could not be established. Other studies [25] concluded that there was no correlation between the occurrence of aggressive affect and psychomotor attacks. When other important factors, like neurological deficits [40,79] and low IQs [109] are controlled, no clear relationship emerges between temporal lobe epilepsy and violence or aggression. Using the Minnesota Multiphasic Inventory, Hermann et al [51] drew a similar conclusion that seizure type was not related to aggression. Using the "TLE Personality Scales" of Bear and Fedio [7], Hermann and Riel [50] found no clear evidence of relationship between aggression and seizure type. Thus, all of these studies failed to establish an increased incidence of violence in patients with epilepsy in general, and temporal lobe epilepsy in particular. It is also possible that the incidence of violence in epileptics is similar to the incidence of violence in the general population.

Further discussion is needed on this controversy of whether there is any *direct* relationship between epilepsy and psychiatric disturbance. The leading advocate against a direct relationship has been Stevens [113] who has summarized the data on this question. She has agreed that patients with major and psychomotor epilepsy are subject to an increased risk of psychiatric disturbances, but that the risk reflects the site and extent of brain damage and the individual's psychosocial history more than it does the diagnosis of epilepsy. She found that EEG abnormalities, usually temporal, were more frequent in patients with violent behavior, schizophrenia, and behavior disorders. However, abnormalities like theta rhythms may reflect a disturbance in the suppression of hippocampal arousal rather than a specific temporal lobe pathology or epilepsy. Furthermore, Stevens [113] adds that the majority of patients with epilepsy, including psychomotor epilepsy, do not develop personality disorders or psychosis. Any psychological disturbance probably relates more to the interactions between environmental causes and the neurological disorders underlying the epilepsy. Hermann and Whitman [49] have more recently summarized the data by stating that in every instance in which direct and indirect data are available, the findings support a relationship between psychosocial variables (not epilepsy) and psychopathology.

In 1975, Waxman and Geschwind claimed that a distinct syndrome of interictal behavior changes was often seen in patients with temporal lobe epilepsy [124]. These changes included alterations in sexual behavior, religiosity, and compulsive writing and drawing. These investigators claimed that it was the interictal spike activity in the temporal structures which provided the pathophysiological basis for this syndrome, exemplifying a human behavioral syndrome associated with dysfunction at specific anatomic loci. Bear and Fedio [7] added more details of these traits, including humorless sobriety, dependence, and obsessions. Patients with a right temporal focus displayed emotional tendencies and denial in contrast to the ideational traits of the patients with left temporal foci, also showing a "catastrophic" overemphasis of dissocial behavior. More recently, various investigators have argued that the latter studies did not exercise sufficiently strict controls on certain variables, thereby invalidating the findings [98].

Violence in the Ictal State

Evidence for violence in the interictal state has been somewhat meager, but an even more important question concerns the ictal state. Since many murderers *claim* to have no memory for their heinous crimes, defense attorneys will often maintain that the "blackout" or memory loss implies a seizure state. Such a condition implies a diminished or absent legal responsibility and introduces a crucial medico-legal question. Delgado-Escueta [27] and later Treiman and Delgado-Escueta [119] have published a list of epilepsy cases used in defense in violent crime cases reaching the U.S. Court of Appeals (data from A.K. Finucane, Epilepsy Foundation of America). From 1889 until 1979, there were 14 such cases and in the 1977 to 1980 period, 11 other cases have made the headlines by attributing murder to an epileptic condition [119].

Examples of actual cases reported in U.S. courts include *Taylor vs United States* [m] adjudicated in 1895. The accused entered a plea of not guilty by reason of insanity. The defense reasoning was (1) a number of psychomotor seizures had caused a state of insanity, (2) a seizure had caused a change of latent insanity to active insanity, and (3) the criminal act had actually transpired during a seizure. The court rejected this defense for lack of evidence that the state of seizure (or activated insanity) adhered to the McNaghten Rules required for the judicial recognition of insanity. In another case, *Oburn vs State* [n] from 1910, the defense was that epilepsy had caused the accused to become insane and that the criminal act, while not occurring during a seizure, was performed by an insane epileptic. The court rejected this defense on the same ground as in the Taylor case: lack of compliance with the McNaghten Rules.

The term *automatism* has also found its way into the courts and was defined in 1961 in *Bratty vs Attorney General for Northern Ireland* [o]. Automatism was considered to be the state of a person who, though capable of action, "is not conscious of what he is doing...It means unconscious involuntary action and it is a defense because the mind does not go with what is being done." Furthermore, automatism "means an act which is done by the muscles without any control by the mind such as a spasm, reflex action or a convulsion; or an act done by a person who is not conscious of what he is doing." Automatism was described in New Zealand in 1958 in *The Queen vs Cottle* [p] as "action without any knowledge of acting, or action with no consciousness of doing what was being done." According to the 1954 decision of the Supreme Court of California in *People vs Baker* [q], "Unconsciousness is a complete, not a partial, defense to a criminal charge." The state of consciousness referred to here is a condition experienced by a normal sane individual wherein "there is no functioning of the conscious mind." *People vs Freeman* [r] pointed out in 1943, "No principle of criminal jurisprudence was ever more zealously guarded than that a person is guiltless if at the time of his commission of an act defined as criminal he has no knowledge of his deed. A person who cannot comprehend the nature and quality of his act is not responsible therefore. An act done in the absence of will is not any more behavior of the actor than is an act done contrary to his will."

Treiman and Delgado-Escueta [119] have compiled the details of 29 cases of acts of aggression or violence allegedly due to an epileptic seizure. Cases include three from East [31] which involve amnesia for the abnormal behavior, including strangling, apparent kidnapping, and post-ictal confusion. A case was described of a murderer who had seizures at ages 2 and 11 years but none for 11 years before and none after the murder, for which the patient claimed amnesia. Another case involved a murder for which at first the patient claimed amnesia but later remembered details. Walker [122] discussed a man who did have complex partial seizures and claimed amnesia during the stabbing of his wife. Although he became hostile during his later seizures and a glioma was discovered in the right temporal lobe, the possibility that his violent act was committed during an ictal state was not clear and not proven. Walker also described a patient who had monthly convulsions and had savagely killed his sisters, possibly in a post-ictal state. MacDonald [72] referred to two patients with seizures who had committed murder, one killing an individual for whom there was great resentment and the other committing the violence in a possible post-ictal state. Other cases include one described by Knox [67] in which aggressive behavior was demonstrated only during attempted restraint of the patient at the end of a psychomotor attack. Gunn and Fenton [43,44] studied 17 cases among 158 seizure patients in the Broadmoor Hospital for the Criminally Insane. One was assaultive, possibly in a post-ictal or drunken state, and in another alcoholic there was no amnesia for the violence. Still another patient became violent only during attempts of restraint while in a post-ictal confusional state. In another case, focal seizures, emotional lability, and episodes of aggressive behavior were often noted, but a direct relationship between the latter symptoms and signs was unclear. In the other 11 cases, premeditation was clear, although seizures had occurred 12 hours before or after the crime. Gunn [41] had one more patient who had epilepsy and killed his wife, but the violence was not witnessed and the patient claimed amnesia for the event.

Banay [5] described four cases of violence possibly related to a seizure, but one could have been an alcoholic intoxication and the other three had psychiatric histories suggestive of an episodic dyscontrol syndrome and violent behavior precipitated by conflicts. In the case described by Stevenson [115], drinking alcohol led to breaking and entering. Because of a left temporal EEG focus, a seizure state was considered to explain this altered behavior. Brewer [12] described a patient who killed two relatives and then became incoherent. Since the EEG showed sharp waves on the right temporal area, psychomotor epilepsy was diagnosed. Milne [80] described a man who murdered his mother after he had been treated for depression and inadequate personality, but had some slow waves and spikes on the right temporal area. He was acquitted since defense counsel argued that the violent attack was that of epileptic automatism. Cope and Donovan [19] reported a patient who had tingling episodes affecting his right arm, at times followed by unprovoked violence. On one occasion he suddenly became aware that he had stabbed a total stranger in the street. Although his EEG was normal, he had an astrocytoma of the left frontal area. Similarly, Simon and DeSilva [106] described a man with episodes of depersonalization and olfactory hallucinations. During an episode he killed his wife, and he was later found to have a tuberculoma of the right frontal lobe.

Perhaps a few cases presented by Mark and Ervin [74] in their book *Violence and the Brain* constitute evidence that a seizure state *might* exist during violent behavior. The case of Mary represents one such possibility: she had had generalized seizures and temporal lobe epilepsy during a 10 year period and had suffered a great personality change with fits of gloom. Her seizures had become more elaborate, and in one instance, the patient attempted repeatedly to stab her husband. From implanted electrodes within the amygdala, "seizure-like" activity was recorded. After electrolytic destruction of the left amygdala, the patient still experienced seizures, but there were no more rage attacks. In the case of Clara, who had a history of head injury and who assaulted nearly anyone who came near her, an electrolytic lesion eliminated the episodes of rage but not all of the seizures. In these instances the authors point out that there is a separation of the episodes of rage from the epileptic attacks, with the latter continuing and the former disappearing after a lesion is placed within the limbic system. Also, there is the case of Thomas who had rage attacks in addition to some typical temporal lobe seizures. Stimulation through an implanted electrode within the limbic system produced a loss of control on the part of the patient. An electrolytic lesion had also eliminated further rage attacks.

Perhaps the most convincing evidence of the *possible* relationship of temporal lobe epilepsy to violent behavior is found in the case of Julia who, at one time, attacked a girl with a sharp instrument and actually pierced the heart of that victim [74]. Spikes were found on the temporal lobe during a routine EEG; with implanted electrodes Mark and Ervin recorded epileptic activity from both amygdalae. Stimulation of the amygdala resulted in symptoms similar to those at the beginning of her clinical seizures. In one instance, clear seizure activity was recorded within the amygdala and at that time, the patient got out of bed, ran to the wall, narrowed her eyes, bared her teeth, clenched her fists, and showed all signs of being on the verge of making an attack. Epileptic activity could be elicited as the result of electrical stimulation through these implanted electrodes, and rage behavior was often seen as the patient attacked the wall. Another time she smashed a guitar against the wall when seizure-like activity was found within the amygdala. At other times, electrical stimulation of the amygdala initiated rage and violence and this behavior was preceded by the development of local electrical seizure activity. The authors stated, "There could be no doubt that the electrical stimulation of and the abnormal seizure activity from the amygdala preceded and was directly related to Julia's violence." This case represents one of the very few instances in the history of epileptology and criminology in which *suggestive* evidence is brought to bear on the question of a possible direct relationship between temporal lobe epilepsy and violent behavior.

Mark and Ervin [74] have also pointed out that certain symptoms of some temporal lobe seizures are very similar to the ones that precede episodes of aggression in violent individuals. However, these authors agree that these instances are not seizures in the usual sense because there is usually no loss of consciousness and no loss of memory for the violent behavior. On the other hand, the episodic violence is said by these authors to reflect a functional abnormality within the temporal lobe. Patients with temporal lobe abnormalities at times share certain behavioral difficulties, including episodes of violence. Most of the individuals studied by Mark and Ervin suffered from *both* seizures and violent episodes. Although temporal lobe epilepsy may be an important example of a known disease state that could possibly be related to violent behavior, these authors are quick to point out that this certainly does not mean that all temporal lobe epileptics are violent. Their belief is that temporal lobe disease can cause a number of conditions, including seizures, severe memory loss, speech difficulty, and poor impulse control including violent behavior. The underlying malfunctioning of the limbic brain is causally related to the poor impulse control and the violent behavior. The temporal lobe seizures represent *only one* symptom of a malfunctioning limbic system [74].

In many of the other cases presented in this section, suggestive evidence exists that a violent episode could have occurred during an ictal (seizure) state. However, in some instances premeditation had occurred; in others, a definite seizure before or after the violence could have been coincidental. These cases indicate episodes provoked by identifiable external stimuli, some related to alcohol intoxication or various kinds of psychiatric states. In the opinion of Treiman and Delgado-Escueta [119], only two cases of Gunn and Fenton [43] and one of Knox [67] provide some evidence of a relationship between ictal events and violent automatisms. However, these were probably in post-ictal confusional states in response to an attempt to restrain the patient.

A newer approach to this problem has been to record a seizure not only on the EEG but also on closed circuit television. Rodin [97] had recorded such ictal events in 150 patients, including 42 psychomotor automatisms, but none showed significant aggressive behavior. Later, King and Ajmone-Marsan [65] checked for violence in 270 epileptic patients with temporal lobe foci, including 199 ictal events. In nine patients, peri-ictal events could be described as somewhat violent, but seven of these patients showed some combativeness during the post-ictal state only with attempts to restrain them and the other two were ineffective in their aggressive acts. Delgado-Escueta et al [28,29] studied 111 patients, but no episodes of aggression directed against a person were observed in 691 seizures recorded on closed circuit TV.

A recent report [30] argues strongly against the probability that violence and epilepsy have any strong connection. Representatives of 16 epilepsy programs from the United States, Canada, Germany, Italy, and Japan selected 19 patients believed to have aggressive behavior during seizures from a group of approximately 5400 patients with epilepsy. Of these 19 patients, 33 attacks were studied and 13 patients had an incontestable diagnosis of epilepsy. Videotape was used to study the seizures of these patients, and values of 0 (no aggressive movement) to 6 (severe violence directed against a person) were used to grade the degree of violence demonstrated on the tape. Six patients scored values of 0 or 1, the remaining seven scored at the values of 2 to 4, representing the only examples of aggressive behavior found in over 5400 patients. Of the seven patients with values of 2 to 4, five had histories of psychiatric or personality disorders; three directed their behavior against inanimate objects; two demonstrated only shouting and spitting; and one showed nondirected aggression. Only the last patient exhibited "violent" behavior against a person, and this action was characterized mainly by scratching of the face, Thus, the authors concluded that only one patient "had aggressive acts that could have resulted in serious harm to another person." A retrospective study of the violent assaults in these patients' life histories revealed that they occurred during kicking or flailing defensive motions, during acts of flight, and in response to being held down or restrained. This international panel suggested five relevant criteria to determine whether a violent crime was the result of an epileptic seizure: (1) the diagnosis of epilepsy should be firmly established by a neurologist skilled in epileptology, (2) epileptic automatisms should be documented by closed-circuit TV and EEG telemetry, (3) any aggressive acts during these automatisms should be verified on videotape with ictal EEG patterns, (4) the violent act should be characteristic of that patient's seizure, and (5) a clinical judgment should be made by a neurologist that the given act was part of a seizure.

Walker [107,122] long ago outlined certain similar criteria that are required to establish that a given crime may have been committed as a manifestation of a seizure. These six criteria were (1) that the patient has bona fide epileptic abnormalities, (2) that spontaneous attacks are similar to the one that occurred at the time of the crime, (3) that the period of the loss of awareness is commensurate with the type of epileptic attack usually experienced by the patient or defendant, (4) that the degree of assumed unconsciousness is commensurate with the degree of unconsciousness with previous attacks, (5) that the EEG findings are compatible with a seizure disorder, and (6) that the circumstances are compatible with the assumption of lack of awareness by the individual at the time of the crime. These six criteria would be very difficult, if not impossible, to establish and relate a violent crime to a seizure disorder.

The findings of the international panel should have the effect of decreasing the number of legal cases attempting to explain violence by a seizure state, since evidence for a close relationship between violence and seizures was found to be very meager [30]. Some have viewed the evidence differently [90] and stated that "this study has amassed convincing clinical evidence that directed violence may be an ictal phenomenon" [30]. Further evidence for the major theme in this section comes from Ramani and Gumnit [94] who studied 19 epileptic patients with a history of episodic aggressive behavior subjected to intensive monitoring. Only two patients actually showed episodic aggressive behavior, but in neither case could seizures be implicated causally. Their conclusion was consistent with the international panel [30] that ictal aggressive behavior, when seen in epileptics, is a multifactorially determined inter-ictal phenomenon.

The questionable phenomenon of "alcohol activation" of the EEG in criminals is relevant to this discussion. A few authors have attempted to document a definite increase in EEG abnormalities, especially epileptiform activity, after ingestion of alcohol, to provide evidence for a possible seizure disorder manifesting as violence after alcohol. However, careful inspection of the evidence [4,73,75,117] has not convinced this author that alcohol produced an epileptic state accounting for the history of violent criminal behavior. After interpreting many EEGs of prisoners given the same amount and type of alcohol that they had ingested before committing a crime, only questionable EEG changes have occurred in very rare instances, and those rare cases have shown no more than slight increases in slow wave abnormalities. Epileptiform activity, like spikes or sharp waves that have rarely appeared after the alcohol, has been the result of the alcohol producing a sleep state which of course is usually required to detect these spikes. Their absence before the alcohol activation has been only that a sleep record had not been achieved in the prior tracing. Even in these few cases, a nonspecific change of a few slow waves does not establish that the abnormal behavior was based on organic brain damage.

As a general conclusion for this section, the author would agree with Whitman et al [129] that "There is thus no basis for defense efforts that suggest that epilepsy is the cause of crime... To deny the conclusions supported by the data is to perpetuate myth and stigma against people with epilepsy and to obscure the role of important social factors."

Other Criminal Acts During Seizures

Morse [82] indicated that when a criminal act, not of aggressiveness or violence, is committed during a psychomotor seizure, there may be another kind of problem of legal responsibility. In 1954 in *Smith vs Commonwealth* [s] an individual with seizures was prosecuted for manslaughter during the operation of an automobile. The defense was that the accused ran over a pedestrian due to a lapse of consciousness which he experienced as a result of the psychomotor seizure. In this case, the jury determined that the accused displayed willful indifference to the safety of other individuals by operating an automobile with knowledge that he had epilepsy. Although the conviction was later reversed because of errors in jury instruction, a subsequent conviction was affirmed in 1955. In the *People vs Freeman* decision [r] consideration was given to the question of whether or not, at the time the accused took to the highway in his automobile, his epileptic condition permitted him to be fully cognizant of what he was doing. The answer was in the negative and the accused was not be held accountable.

The sum and substance of the Smith decision [s] seems to be that an individual with epilepsy who has had at least one prior seizure drives an automobile distinctly at his own criminal risk. The Smith decision may appear to be more reasonable than the Freeman decision, since the safety of the public and the consideration for potential automobile accident victims should certainly outweigh the importance of an individual's driving privilege [82]. The reviewer agrees with this general point.

Limitation of EEG in the Courtroom

Pessimism has been expressed by a number of authors regarding the usefulness of the EEG in the courtroom. For example, Kiloh and Osselton [64] reported that in forensic psychiatry, electroencephalography, with its shades of value and relatively low scale of probability, finds little application. They point to two cases of murder discussed by Curran [24]. In both cases, the EEG showed quite obvious abnormalities – one patient with spike and wave activity and the other with changes suggestive of a localized brain lesion. However, there was no clinical evidence to support a diagnosis of epilepsy in either case, and in both instances the crimes seemed to be described as calculated and purposive. It was argued at both trials that the EEG abnormalities indicated the presence of "brain pathology" relevant to the commission of the crimes. These arguments were discarded by both juries and subsequent necropsy of the brain in each case proved to be normal.

Perr [86] summarized the evidence on the limitations of EEG in the courtroom and found that EEG findings following injury are of little prognostic significance. This general statement must make the electroencephalographer cautious about his predictions in a court of law. Furthermore, Walton [123] indicated that he had given up using EEG in medico-legal cases. He did point out, however, that although a single EEG in head injury cases is of little diagnostic or prognostic value, serial recordings are useful in expressing the likelihood that post-traumatic epilepsy will develop. Clinical experience, rather than the EEG alone, was what Walton relied upon in these instances. In the case of the *State vs Carlson* [t], EEG tracings were presented as showing an organic abnormality in a defendant charged with arson. However, since no other information regarding organic changes was presented in this case, the court held that the electroencephalographic tracings stood alone without any further expert medical testimony and were of no probative value. This reviewer does not share the pessimism of these latter authors since there are many trials in which EEG has played a prominent and proper role. The recurring symposia on legal EEG also demonstrate that this test continues to properly find its way into many court cases.

Practical Suggestions for Medico-Legal Cases

Gibbs and Gibbs [34] offer some excellent suggestions for the electroencephalographer about to appear in court. They point out that the electroencephalographer is likely to receive telephone calls from lawyers of both sides and even possibly from the patient or members of the family. Obviously, the physician must be extremely careful about imparting information, especially to the "other side." Gibbs and Gibbs point out that legal proceedings are usually tedious, especially when the electroencephalographer may need to spend an entire day waiting without being called to the stand. They further point out that on the succeeding day one may be forced to spend many more hours conveying a small amount of information which would have required only a few words if one were allowed to state them "in a normal manner." This reviewer would strongly suggest that appointments made between the electroencephalographer and the lawyer for a court appearance should be for the earliest possible hour in the morning, usually 10 o'clock. Under these circumstances one usually can get on the witness stand near the beginning of the morning session; but if one waits for the afternoon for a scheduled first appearance, delays of the morning usually mean a long wait before being called to the witness stand.

The Gibbses [34] point out that science and law do not mix and that "lawsuits seem to be a survival from a prescientific era, a kind of trial by combat." They point out that both sides distort the evidence as much as they can and that the lawyers on both sides attempt to cajole, trick, or actually frighten witnesses into saying what they do not mean to say. The reviewer would generally agree with these latter points. Also, Gibbs and Gibbs point out that lawyers commonly indulge in forms of unpleasantness that are rarely encountered outside a courtroom. Normal procedure in the court may also involve disparaging comments regarding the intelligence, competence, and probity of the witness. The attorney responsible for the court appearance of the electroencephalographer must take care to safeguard that person's reputation. The Gibbses conclude that electroencephalographers should not feel they have been singled out for special abuse, if handled roughly, since nearly every witness may receive the same kind of treatment. To be prepared, be sure to have a detailed pretrial discussion with the attorney who has called you to court. Each and every question to be asked of you, the electroencephalographer, in court should be written out by the attorney and the answer to each of these questions should be clear to you. Often the electroencephalographer must instruct the attorney about the kinds of questions to ask that directly relate to the EEG. Many attorneys are somewhat knowledgeable of electroencephalography, but most will require some help from the electroencephalographer in formulating good questions to prepare a case either that a given record is normal or that it shows certain abnormalities.

One further point is very important. During cross-examination the electroencephalographer should try to foresee the direction the opposing attorney is taking, to avoid being led into traps. Be aware that a yes or no answer to questions can be misleading to everyone in the courtroom, including the jury; thus, if you think questions requiring yes-no answers are leading judge and jury to incorrect conclusions, you should request permission from the judge to explain the answers in greater detail. The Gibbses also refer to this problem and point out that the witness is asked to subscribe to the legal fiction that the truth can be extracted through questions that are answered simply yes or no, but that one is required under oath to tell the *whole* truth and nothing but the truth. They also point out that electroencephalographers as witnesses must be aware that their answers may be adding up to a total falsehood and that they should turn to the judge and indicate that they must be able to explain further and in greater detail. In my experience, most judges permit one to provide such details. As Gibbs and Gibbs point out, neither the plaintiff's attorney nor the attorney for the defense may be really interested in the truth as the electroencephalographer sees it, but it is important for the EEG witness to present testimony clearly and in the most accurate way.

The Gibbses [34] also point out that various well-known tricks are often used by attorneys during cross-examination concerning the EEG. These include statements that most brain-wave abnormalities are really meaningless, either because they occur in persons who are perfectly normal or else because they can be caused by "anything." Another common trick is to declare the EEG inadmissible because the electroencephalographer did not see the patient at the time of the recording. The usual absence of the electroencephalographer during the recording should be brought out by the opposing attorney, but if not, the electroencephalographer must quickly add (whenever possible) that our presence is rarely required during most recordings. One of the subtlest tricks, commonly used in cross-examination, is for the opposing attorney to use terms with a questionable definition and ask for agreement regarding some statement incorporating those terms. The witness who has agreed to a number of these statements may suddenly realize that the points add up to a conclusion opposite to the previously stated position. The important point is to request and require a precise definition from the attorney who uses a term that has a questionable definition. This maneuver puts the attorney on the defensive and reverses what they are trying to accomplish with the witness. Gibbs and Gibbs point out that it is helpful to remember that the other attorney is going to try to "get your goat" and that supposedly there are no hard feelings afterward.

To conclude, what the electroencephalographer needs most in court is a positive attitude. If the attorney and electroencephalographer-witness have carefully planned their scenario and each knows what the other will be saying, then the only problem that remains will be the cross-examination from the opposing attorney. Here a positive attitude is required in which the physicians must forever be aware of their stated position in the case, must try to foresee how the other attorney is attempting to shake their testimony, and should consider these verbal interchanges as an interesting intellectual challenge. After all, we should know our business better than any attorney and should triumph in all or most of these intellectual combats if we remain calm or cool. With a positive attitude of this sort, the reviewer has actually enjoyed most courtroom appearances and has found them to be fascinating experiences.

REFERENCES

1. Aird RB, Masland RL, Woodbury DM. The Epilepsies: A Critical Review, New York, Raven Press, 1984.

2. Alstrom CH, 1950. A study of epilepsy in its clinical, social, and genetic aspects. Copenhagen, Ejnar Munksgaard, 1950.

3. Ascroft PB. Traumatic epilepsy after gunshot wounds of the head. Brit Med J, 1941, 1:739-744.

4. Bach-y-Rita G, Lion JR, Ervin FR. Pathological intoxication: clinical and electroencephalographic studies. Am J Psychiat, 1970, 127:698-702.

5. Banay RS. Criminal genesis and the degree of responsibility in epilepsies. Am J Psychiat, 1961, 117:873-876.

6. Baumann RJ, Marx MB, Leonidakis MG. Epilepsy in rural Kentucky: prevalence in a population of school age children. Epilepsia, 1978, 19:75-80.

7. Bear DM, Fedio P. Quantitative analysis of interictal behavior in temporal lobe epilepsy. Arch Neurol, 1977, 34:454-467.

8. Birkmayer W. Die behandlung der tramatischen epilepsie. Wien Klin Wochenschr, 1951, 63:606-609.

9. Blackwood D, McQueen JK, Harris P, et al. A clinical trial of phenytoin in the prophylaxis of epilepsy following head injury: A preliminary report. In: Dam M, Gram L, Penry JK (eds), Advances in Epileptology: 12th Epilepsy International Symposium. New York, Raven Press, 1981.

10. Bluglass RS. A Psychiatric Study of Scottish Prisoners. Unpublished MD Thesis, 1966. Cited by Gunn, 1977.

11. Bouzarth WF, Goldman HW. Prophylactic phenytoin. J Neurosurg, 1984, 59:877.

12. Brewer C. Homicide during a psychomotor seizure. Med J Austria, 1971, 857-859.

13. Brewis M, Poskanzer D, Rolland C, Miller H. Neurological disease in an English city. Acta Neurol Scand, 1966, 42(Suppl 24):1-89.

14. Burt C. The Young Delinquent. London, UCP, 1944.

15. Caveness WF. Onset and cessation of fits following craniocerebral trauma. J Neurosurg, 1963, 20:570-583.

16. Caveness WF. Epilepsy, a product of trauma in our time. Epilepsia, 1976, 17:207-215.

17. Caveness WF, Meirowsky AM, Rish BL, et al. The nature of posttraumatic epilepsy. J Neurosurg, 1979, 50:545-553.

18. Chiafalo N, Kirschbaum A, Fuentes A, et al. Prevalence of epilepsy in children of Melipilla, Chile. Epilepsia, 1979, 20:261-266.

19. Cope RV, Donovan WM. A case of insane automatism? Brit J Psychiat, 1979, 135:574-575.

20. Courjon JA. Post-traumatic epilepsy in electro-clinical practice. In: Walker AE, Caveness WF, Critchley M (eds), Late Effects of Head Injury. Springfield IL, Charles C Thomas, 1969.

21. Courjon J. Apport de l'exploration fonctionelle du systeme nerveux dans le diagnostic et le pronostic des traumatismes craniens recents. Acta Neurol Belg, 1970, 70:359-377.

22. Courjon J. Handbook of Electroencephalography and Clinical Neurophysiology, vol 14B, Traumatic Disorders. Amsterdam, Elsevier, 1972.

23. Cowie J, Cowie V, Slater E. Delinquency in Girls. London, Heinemann, 1968.

24. Curran D. Psychiatry Ltd. J Ment Sci, 1952, 98:373-381.

25. Currie S, Heathfield KWG, Henson RA, Scott DF. Clinical course and prognosis of temporal lobe epilepsy. Brain, 1971, 94:173-190.

26. Credner L. Klinische und sociale Auswerkungen von Hirnschadigungen. Z Gesamte Neurol Psychiat, 1930, 126:721-757.

27. Delgado-Escueta AV. Seizure disorder update, vol 2, The illusion of violence in epilepsy. Parke-Davis, Warner-Lambert, 1981, pp 19-28.

28. Delgado-Escueta AV, Bacsal FE, Treiman DM. Complex partial seizures on closed-circuit television and EEG: A study of 691 attacks in 79 patients. Ann Neurol, 1982, 11:292-300.

29. Delgado-Escueta AV, Kunze U, Waddell G, et al. Lapse of consciousness and automatisms in temporal lobe epilepsy: a videotape analysis. Neurology (Minneap), 1977, 27:144-155.

30. Delgado-Escueta AV, Mattson RH, King L, Goldensohn ES, Spiegel H, Madsen J, Crandall P, Dreifuss F, Porter RJ. Special report. The nature of aggression during epileptic seizures. New Engl J Med, 1981, 305:711-716.

31. East WN. An introduction to forensic psychiatry in the criminal courts. New York, Williams Wood & Company, 1927.

32. Gibbens TCN, Prince J. Shoplifting. London, ISTD, 1962.

33. Gibbs FA, Gibbs EL. Atlas of Electroencephalography, vol 2. Reading MA, Addison-Wesley, 1952.

34. Gibbs FA, Gibbs EL. Atlas of Electroencephalography, vol 3. Reading MA, Addison-Wesley, 1964.

35. Gibbs FA, Bloomberg W, Bagchi BK. Electroencephalographic study of criminals. Amer J Psychiat, 1945, 102:294-298.

36. Gibbs FA, Weigner WR, Gibbs EL. The electroencephalogram in post-traumatic epilepsy. Amer J Psychiat, 1944, 100:738-749.

37. Gomez JG, Arciniegas E, Torres J. Prevalence of epilepsy in Bogota, Columbia. Neurology, 1978, 28:90-94.

38. Gotze W, Wolter M. Grenzen der Hirnstromuntersuchung bei der Begutachtung von Hirntraumafolgen. Med Sachverst, 1957, 53:104-109.

39. Gudmundsson G. Epilepsy in Ireland, a clinical and epidemiological investigation. Acta Neurol Scand (Suppl 25), 1966, 43:1-124.

40. Guerrant J, Anderson WW, Fischer A, et al. Personality in Epilepsy. Springfield IL, Charles C Thomas, 1962.

41. Gunn J. Epileptics in Prison. London, Academic Press, 1977.

42. Gunn J, Bonn J. Criminality and violence in epileptic prisoners. Brit J Psychiat, 1971, 118:337-343.

43. Gunn J, Fenton G. Epilepsy in prisons, a diagnostic survey. Brit Med J, 1969, 4:326.

44. Gunn J, Fenton G. Epilepsy, automatism and crime. Lancet, 1971, 1:1173-1176.

45. Hagan CA. The insanity defense. J Legal Med, 1982, 3:617-647.

46. Hauser WA, Kurland LT. The epidemiology of epilepsy in Rochester, Minnesota, 1935 through 1967. Epilepsia, 1975, 16:1-66.

47. Healy W. The individual delinquent. Boston, Little Brown & Co, 1929.

48. Hendrick EB, Harris L. Post-traumatic epilepsy in children. J Trauma, 1968, 8:547.

49. Hermann BP, Whitman S. Psychopathology in epilepsy. A multietiological model. In: Whitman S, Hermann BP (eds), Psychopathology in Epilepsy. New York, Oxford, 1986, pp 5-37.

50. Hermann BP, Riel P. Interictal personality and behavioral traits in temporal lobe and primary generalized epilepsy. Cortex, 1981, 17:125-128.

51. Hermann BP, Schwartz MS, Whitman S, Karnes WE. Aggression and epilepsy: seizure type comparisons and high risk variables. Epilepsia, 1980, 22:691-698.

52. Hill D. EEG in episodic, psychotic and psychopathic behavior, a classification of data. Electroencephalogr Clin Neurophysiol, 1952, 4:419-442.

53. Hill D, Pond DA. Reflections on one hundred capital cases admitted to electroencephalography. J Ment Sci, 1952, 98:23-43.

54. Hollingsworth JS. Mental retardation, cerebral palsy and epilepsy in Alabama. Tuscaloosa AL, University of Alabama, 1978.

55. Hyslop GH. Seizures, head injuries and litigants. Indust Hyg Toxicol, 1949, 31:336-342.

56. James IP. Temporal lobectomy for psychomotor epilepsy. J Ment Sci, 1960, 106:543-558.

57. Jasper H, Penfield W. Electroencephalograms in post-traumatic epilepsy. Amer J Psychiat, 1943, 100:365-377.

58. Jennett B. Early traumatic epilepsy. Arch Neurol, 1974, 30:394-398.

59. Jennett B. Epilepsy after Non-missile Head Injuries, ed 2. Chicago, Year Book Medical, 1975.

60. Jennett B, Teasdale G. Management of Head Injuries. Philadelphia, FA Davis Co, 1981.

164   *John R. Hughes*

61. Johnson AL, Harris P, McQueen JK, et al. Phenytoin prophylaxis for post-traumatic seizures. J Neurosurg, 1984, 59:727-731.
62. Jung R. Neurophysiologische Untersuchungsmethoden. In: Von Bergmann G, Frey W, Schwiegk H, (eds), Handbuch der Inneren Medizin, vol 1. Berlin, Springer, 1953, pp 1206-1420.
63. Kennard MA, Rabinovitch MS, Fister WP. The use of frequency analysis in the interpretation of EEGs of patients with psychological disorders. Electroencephalogr Clin Neurophysiol, 1955, 7:29-38.
64. Kiloh LG, Osselton JW. Clinical Electroencephalography. London, Butterworth, 1961.
65. King DW, Ajmone Marsan C. Clinical features and ictal patterns in epileptic patients with EEG temporal lobe foci. Ann Neur, 1977, 2:138-147.
66. King LM, Young QD. Increased prevalence of seizure disorders among prisoners. JAMA, 1978, 239:2674-2675.
67. Knox SJ. Epileptic automatism and violence. Med Sci Law, 1968, 8:96-104.
68. Levy S. A study of the electroencephalogram as related to personality structure in a group of inmates of a state penitentiary. Electroencephalogr Clin Neurophysiol, 1952, 4:113.
69. Levy S, Kennard MA. Study of electroencephalogram as related to personality structure in group of inmates of state penitentiary. Amer J Psychiat, 1953, 109:832-839.
70. Lewis DO. Delinquency, psychomotor epileptic symptoms and paranoid ideation: a triad. Amer J Psychiat, 1976, 133:1395-1398.
71. Lewis DO, Pincus JH, Shanok SS, Glaser GH. Psychomotor epilepsy and violence in a group of incarcerated adolescent boys. Amer J Psychiat, 1982, 139:882-887.
72. MacDonald JM. Psychiatry and the criminal. Springfield IL, Charles C Thomas, 1969.
73. Maletzky BM. The diagnosis of pathological intoxication. J Stud Alcohol, 1976, 37:1215-1288.
74. Mark VH, Ervin FR. Violence and the brain. New York, Harper & Row, 1970.
75. Marinacci AA. Special type of temporal lobe seizures following ingestion of alcohol. Bull Los Angeles Neurol Soc, 1963, 28:241-250.
76. Marshall C, Walker AE. The value of electroencephalography in the prognostication and prognosis of post-traumatic epilepsy. Epilepsia, 1961, 2:138-143.
77. Matheson JCM, Hill D. Electroencephalography in medico-legal problems. Med-Leg Rev, 1943, 11:173-181.
78. Meyer-Mickeleit RW. Das Electroencephalogram nach gedeckten Kopfverletzungen. Dtsch Med Wochenschr, 1953, 1:480-484.
79. Mignone RJ, Donnelly EF, Sadowsky D. Psychological and neurological comparisons of psychomotor and nonpsychomotor epileptic patients. Epilepsia, 1970, 11:345-369.
80. Milne HB. Epileptic homicide: drug induced. Brit J Psychiat, 1979, 134:547-548.
81. Morris T, Blom-Cooper L. A Calendar of Murder. London, Joseph, 1964.
82. Morse HN. The aberrational man—a tour de force of legal psychiatry. J Forensic Sci, 1968, 13:1-13, 365-369, 488-497.
83. Novick LF, Penna RD, Schwartz MS, Remmlinger E, Loewenstein R. Health status of the New York City prison population, Med Care 1977, 15:205-216.
84. O'Connell BA. America and homicide. Brit J Delinq, 1960, 10:262-276.
85. Ounsted C. Aggression and epilepsy rage in children with temporal lobe epilepsy. J Psychosom Res, 1969, 13:237-242.
86. Perr IN. Medico-legal aspects of post-traumatic epilepsy. Amer J Psychiat, 1960, 116:981-992.
87. Penry JK, White BG, Brackett CE. A controlled prospective study of the pharmacologic prophylaxis of post-traumatic epilepsy. Neurology, 1979, 29:600-601.
88. Phillips G. Traumatic epilepsy after closed head injury. J Neurol Neurosurg Psychiat, 1954, 17:1-10.
89. Pincus JH, Lewis DO, Shanok SS, Glaser GH. Neurologic abnormalities in violent delinquents. Neurology, 1979, 29:586.

90. Pincus JH. Can violence be a manifestation of epilepsy? Neurology, 1980, 30:304-307.
91. Pitcher DR. The XYY syndrome. Brit J Psychiat Spec, 1975, 9:316-325.
92. Planques J, Grezes-Rueff CH. L'electroencephalographie dans l'expertise medico-legale. XXVIIeme Congres International de Medecine du Travail. Medecine Legale et Medecine Sociale de Langue Francaise. Strasbourg, A Coueslant, Cahors, 1954.
93. Popek K. Preventive treatment of post-traumatic epilepsy following severe brain injury. Czech Neurol, 1972, 35:35-68.
94. Ramani V, Gumnit R. Intensive monitoring of epileptic patients with a history of episodic aggression. Arch Neurol, 1981, 38:570-571.
95. Riley T, Niedermeyer E. Rage attacks and episodic violent behavior: electroencephalographic findings and general consideration. Clin EEG, 1978, 9:113-139.
96. Rish BL, Caveness WF. Relation of prophylactic medication to the occurrence of early seizures following craniocerebral trauma. J Neurosurg, 1973, 38:155-158.
97. Rodin EA. Psychomotor epilepsy and aggressive behavior. Arch Gen Psychiat, 1973, 28:210-213.
98. Rodin E, Schmaltz S. The Bear-Fedio personality inventory and temporal lobe epilepsy. Epilepsia, 1983, 24:260.
99. Russell WR, Whitty CWM. Studies in traumatic epilepsy: factors influencing incidence of epilepsy after brain wounds. J Neurol Neurosurg Psychiat, 1952, 15:93-98.
100. Scherzer E. Uber die gutachtliche Wertung des 4/sec Rhythmus nach Schadeltraumen. Psychiatr Neurol (Basel), 1965, 150:8-20.
101. Serafetinides EA. Aggressiveness in temporal lobe epileptics and its relation to cerebral dysfunction and environmental factors. Epilepsia, 1965, 6:33-42.
102. Servit Z. Pharmacological prophylaxis of post-traumatic epilepsy – clinical results and theoretical implications. In: Majkowski J (ed), Post-traumatic Epilepsy and Pharmacological Prophylaxis. Warsaw, Poland, International League Against Epilepsy, 1977.
103. Shamansky SL, Glaser GH. Socioeconomic characteristics of disorders in the New Haven area: an epidemiologic study. Epilepsia, 1979, 20:457-474.
104. Silverman D. Clinical and electroencephalographic studies on criminal psychopaths. Arch Neurol Psychiat, 1943, 50:18-33.
105. Silverman D. The electroencephalogram of criminals. Arch Neurol Psychiat, 1944, 52:38-42.
106. Simon RH, Desilva M. Intracranial tuberculoma coexistent with uncinate seizures and violent behavior. JAMA, 1981, 245:1247-1248.
107. Southern EEG Society. Electroencephalography and the law, Moot trial proceedings on two cases. Birmingham AL, 1968.
108. Small JG. The organic dimension of crime. Arch Gen Psychiat, 1966, 15:82-89.
109. Small JG, Small IF, Hayden MP. Further psychiatric investigations of patients with temporal and non-temporal lobe epilepsy. Amer J Psychiat, 1966, 123:303-310.
110. Stafford-Clark D, Taylor FH. Clinical and electroencephalographic studies of prisoners charged with murder. J Neurol Neurosurg Psychiat, 1949, 12:325-330.
111. Stafford-Clark D, Pond D, Lovett Doust JW. The psychopath in prison: a preliminary report of a co-operative research. Brit Delinq, 1951, 2:117-129.
112. Stevens JR. An anatomy of schizophrenia? Arch Gen Psychiat, 1973, 29:177-189.
113. Stevens JR. Interictal clinical manifestations of complex partial seizures. In: Penry JK, Daly DD (eds), Advances in Neurology, vol 11, New York, Raven, 1975, pp 85-112.
114. Stevens JR, Hermann BP. Temporal lobe epilepsy, psychopathology, and violence: the state of the evidence. Neurology, 1981, 31:1127-1132.
115. Stevenson HG. Psychomotor epilepsy associated with criminal behavior. Med Austria, 1963, 50:784-785.
116. Terespolsky PS. Post-traumatic epilepsy. Forensic Sci, 1972, 1:147-165.

117. Thompson GN. The electroencephalogram in acute pathological alcoholic intoxication. Bull Los Angeles Neurol Soc, 1963, 28:217-224.
118. Treiman DM, Delgado Escueta AV. Aggression during fear and flight in complex partial seizures: A CCTV-EEG analysis. Epilepsia, 1981, 22:243.
119. Treiman DM, Delgado-Escueta AV. Violence and epilepsy: a critical review. In: Pedley TA, Meldrum BA (eds), Recent Advances in Epilepsy. New York, Churchill-Livingstone, 1983, pp 179-210.
120. Vogel F. Genetische Aspekte des Electroencephalograms. Dtsch Med Wochenschr, 1963, 88:1748-1759.
121. Walker AE. Pathogenesis and pathophysiology of post traumatic epilepsy. In: Walker AE, Caveness WR, Critchley M (eds), The Late Effects of Head Injury. Springfield IL, Charles C Thomas, 1969.
122. Walker AE. Murder or epilepsy? J Nerv Ment Dis, 1961, 133:430-437.
123. Walton JN. Some observations on the value of electroencephalography in medico-legal practice. Medicoleg J, 1963, 31:15-35.
124. Waxman SG, Geschwind N. The interictal behavior syndrome of temporal lobe epilepsy. Arch Gen Psychiat, 1975, 32:1580-1586.
125. Weiss GH, Caveness WF. Prognostic factors in the persistence of post-traumatic epilepsy. J Neurosurg, 1972, 37:164-169.
126. Weiss GH, Salazar AM, Vance SC, et al. Predicting post-traumatic epilepsy in penetrating head injury. Arch Neurol, 1986, 43:771-773.
127. West DJ. The Habitual Prisoner. London, Heinemann, 1963.
128. Whitman S, Coleman T, Berg B, et al. Epidemiological insights into the socioeconomic correlates of epilepsy. In: Hermann B (ed), A Multidisciplinary Handbook of Epilepsy. Springfield IL, Charles C Thomas, 1980, pp 243-271.
129. Whitman S, King LN, Cohen RL. Epilepsy and violence: A scientific and social analysis. In: Whitman S, Hermann BP (eds), Psychopathology in Epilepsy. New York, Oxford Univ Press, 1986, pp 284-302.
130. Whitty CWM. Early traumatic epilepsy. Brain, 1947, 70:416-439.
131. Williams D. Neural factors related to habitual aggression: consideration of differences between those habitual aggressives and others who have committed crimes of violence. Brain, 1969, 92:503-520.
132. Winkler GE, Kove SS. Implications of electroencephalographic abnormalities in homicide cases. Neuropsychiatry, 1962, 3:322-330.
133. Witkin HA, Mednick SA, Schulsinger F, et al. Criminality in XYY and XXY men. Science, 1976, 193:547-555.
134. Wohms RNW, Wyler AR. Prophylactic phenytoin in severe head injuries. J Neurosurg, 1979, 57:507-509.
135. Woolsey RM, Goldner JA. Forensic aspects of electroencephalography. Med Trial Tech Q, 1975, (Winter):338-348.
136. Young B, Rapp R, Brooks WH, et al. Post traumatic epilepsy prophylaxis. Epilepsia, 1979, 20:671-681.
137. Young B, Rapp RP, Norton JA, et al. Failure of prophylactically administered phenytoin to prevent early post-traumatic seizures. J Neurosurg, 1983, 58:231-235.

LEGAL REFERENCES

a. Rex vs McNaghten. 10 Clark and Finnelly 200 (1843).
b. Betz vs Travis Insurance Co., 68 So 2d 669 (La.App., 1953).
c. Melford vs Gaus and Brown Construction Co., 17 Ill. App. 2d 497, 151 N.E. 2d 128 (1958).

d. Annotation: Admissibility in civil action of electroencephalogram, electrocardiogram, or other record made by instrument used in medical test, or of report based upon such test, 66 ALR2d 537 (1959).

e. Croll vs John Hancock Mut. Life Ins. Co., 198 F2d 562 (CA 3rd, 1952).

f. Kramer vs John Hancock Mut. Life Ins. Co., 336 Mass 465, 146 NE2d 357 (1957).

g. Young vs Liddington, 50 Wash2d 78, 309 P2d 761 (1957).

h. Maypole vs Crystal and Son Inc., 266 App Div. 1008, 44 N.Y.S.2d 411, 412 (1943).

i. Quadlander vs Kansas City Public Service Co., 240 Mo App 1134, 224 SW2d 396 (1949).

j. Hinrichs vs Young (Mo), 403 SW2d 642 (1966).

k. Frey vs State, 171 Tex. Crim. 100, 345 S.W.2d 416 (1961).

l. Armstead vs State, 227 Md. 73, 175 A.2d 24 (1961).

m. Taylor vs United States, 7 App. D.C. 27 (1895).

n. Oburn vs State, 143 Wis. 249, 126 N.W. 737 (1910).

o. Bratty vs Attorney General for Northern Ireland, (1961) 3 All E.R. 523, 527, 532, (1963) A.C. 368, 401, 409: (1961) 3 W.L.R. 965, 972, 978, 105, Sol. Jo. 865; 46 Cr. App. Rep. 1, 7, 8, 16, H.L.

p. The Queen vs Cottle, (1958) N.2L.R. 999, 1020.

q. People vs Baker, 42 Cal 2d 550, 575, 268 P.2d 705, 720 (1954).

r. People vs. Freeman, 61 Cal. App. 2d 110, 117, 142, P.2d 435, 439 (Cal. App., 1943).

s. Smith vs Commonwealth, 268 S.W. 2d 937 (Ky., 1954).

t. State vs Carlson, 5 Wis. 2d 595, 93 N.W. 2d 354 (1958).

Chapter 8

Neurobehavioral Outcome
after Closed Head Injury

Felicia C. Goldstein, Harvey S. Levin,
and Howard M. Eisenberg

The neurobehavioral consequences of closed head injury (CHI) consist of alterations in cognitive functioning including general intellectual ability, memory, information processing and language, as well as changes in behavior and psychosocial
adaptation. As investigators have noted, attempts to establish direct brain-behavior
relationships are oversimplistic because variables other than neurologic indices
undoubtedly play a part in the temporal course of recovery [9,14,49,50]. Pre-injury
factors reflecting the emotional stability of the patient and support of the family may
influence the neurobehavioral disturbance beyond the acute stages [5,49,50,65]. In
addition, a higher degree of premorbid education and occupation may impart a
better prognosis for return to work [21,64]. Current environmental conditions such
as the patient's and family's responses to illness also moderate outcome. Depression
may arise from loss and frustration [48] or conversely, the patient may exhibit denial
and resist therapy [63]. Family members can prolong the period of dependence, as
has been suggested with the postconcussional syndrome [77].

Against this background, it is appreciated that the prediction of recovery of
neurobehavioral functioning becomes an exceedingly difficult task. In this chapter,
we review the common sequelae in head-injured adults with a discussion of clinicopathological features and their postulated relationship to outcome. It is

Goldstein, Levin, and Eisenberg

Table 8.1. Frequently Employed Indices and Measures of Neurobehavioral Functioning Following Closed Head Injury

Clinical Indices
Severity and Duration of Impaired Consciousness
Acute Hemiparesis
Oculocephalic/Oculovestibular and Pupillary Responses
Presence/Site of Focal Hemispheric Mass Lesion
Duration of Post-traumatic Amnesia

Neurobehavioral Outcome	
Cognitive Features	**Behavioral Features**
General Intellectual Recovery	Acute Confusional State
Reasoning/Problem Solving	Mood Disturbance
Memory	Insight and Motivational Disturbances
Attention	Somatic Complaints
Language	

highlighted that variables other than the severity of injury, while not always investigated, also contribute to recovery. For reviews of pediatric CHI, the reader is referred to papers by Fletcher et al [17], Goldstein and Levin [22], and Shapiro [71].

NEUROLOGIC INDICES OF INJURY ANALYZED IN STUDIES OF NEUROBEHAVIORAL OUTCOME

Several neurologic indices have been utilized to examine the relationship between acute injury and recovery of cognition and behavior. Table 8.1 outlines the most frequently employed indices and the aspects of neurobehavioral functioning which have been investigated. The Glasgow Coma Scale (GCS) [78], which characterizes the severity and duration of impaired consciousness, has provided a powerful research tool to assist in stratifying patient subgroups. The GCS consists of three dimensions (eye opening, motor and verbal responses) which are rated and summed to provide a composite score of 3 to 15 points. In general, scores of 8 or less define severe injury, 9 to 12 – moderate injury, and 13 to 15 – mild injury. Scores of 8 or less within 24 hours have been found to portend a poor cognitive outcome [1].

The duration of coma is determined through serial assessment and is typically defined as the interval in which there is no eye opening, an inability to obey commands, and absence of speech. However, there is considerable variability across studies in using coma as distinguished from impaired consciousness based on the total GCS score. The motor scale provides almost as powerful a predictor of global outcome as the total sum or the eye and verbal categories alone [33]. Increased standardization across studies employing duration of coma or the period of inability to follow commands will aid in examining the predictive power of this index in relation to outcome.

Acute hemiparesis and integrity of brain stem reflexes including eye movements and pupillary responses have also been utilized to document severity. Hemiparesis following severe CHI does not appear to play a major predictive role in global outcome [34]. In contrast, abnormal brainstem reflexes have been found to contribute to prolonged disability and neuropsychological impairment [1,2,34,42].

Classification of CHI includes the presence and site of a focal hemispheric mass lesion. Diffuse injuries are typically defined by the absence of sizable intracranial lesions on computerized tomographic (CT) scans, whereas focal hemispheric injuries are divided according to their location (left, right, bilateral). Research has demonstrated specific impairments depending upon side of injury (e.g., verbal deficits following dominant left hemisphere lesions; visuospatial deficits following nondominant right hemisphere lesions) and specific area (e.g., memory deficits after temporal lobe lesions) [37,41,80]. In general these relationships are variable, which may be due, in part, to limitations in neuroimaging and the effects of concomitant diffuse injury. Recent reports [19,30,36] have indicated the relative advantage of magnetic resonance imaging (MRI) in detecting intracranial abnormalities undisclosed by CT, particularly with respect to parenchymal and extraparenchymal lesions. In addition, MRI may be better able to capture the size of lesions. Figures 8.1A and 8.1B show CT and MRI scans obtained in a patient with mild CHI five days after injury. The left frontal lobe hematoma was visualized as larger in the MRI scan, and an additional lesion was detected in the left parietal area. Studies examining size and resolution of lesions in relation to neurobehavioral functioning will contribute to an understanding of prediction of outcome.

Post-traumatic amnesia (PTA) [66] consists of a period of confusion and memory loss during which the patient is unable to register day-to-day information including orientation to place and time as well as events following trauma. Injuries that produce coma tend to result in longer periods of PTA but there is considerable variability, even in patients sustaining mild or moderate injuries. Serial assessment of orientation by such measures as the Galveston Orientation and Amnesia Test [47] provides an estimate of PTA duration. The length of PTA has been found to correlate with short term measures of global outcome and cognitive functioning [10,32], with periods of < 2 weeks generally predictive of a better recovery.

The above measures have provided the most consistent means of characterizing patient subgroups. In the following sections, we review the major cognitive and behavioral sequelae of CHI with a consideration of clinical indices related to recovery.

FEATURES OF COGNITIVE RECOVERY

General Intellectual Functioning

Studies examining intellectual recovery have tended to use the Wechsler Adult Intelligence Test (WAIS) [83] or its revised version, the WAIS-R [84]. Researchers have suggested a dissociation in the impairment and recovery of Verbal IQ (e.g., fund

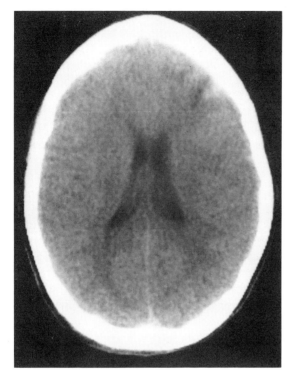

Figure 8.1A. Baseline CT scan obtained five days after injury showing a left frontal lesion, seen as an area of mixed low and high density.

of general information, digit repetition, conceptual reasoning) versus Performance IQ (e.g., arrangement of blocks to form a pattern, puzzle completion, speeded transcription of numbers/symbols) [6,15,42,53]. During the initial stages of 6 to 12 months after moderate or severe CHI, scores on the Verbal Scale level off earlier than for the Performance Scale, indicating that verbal functions may recover more quickly than visuospatial/visuomotor skills [53]. This overall pattern has been proposed to reflect an increased vulnerability of domains such as speed of information processing as opposed to Verbal IQ which tends to be influenced by cultural/educational factors. Studies have also suggested that the general rate of improvement in intellectual functioning slows after the first year following a severe had injury [51,52,53,76]. However, statements regarding potential for further recovery must be made cautiously pending investigations utilizing serial testing, consideration of lateralization factors (e.g., hemispheric mass lesion), and measures of differential recovery slopes.

Investigators have attempted to delineate the clinical variables related to cognitive outcome. Predictors of residual cognitive functioning have included the degree and duration of impaired consciousness [1,10,32,42], presence and neuroanatomic locus of focal hemispheric injury [41,43,80], and oculovestibular and pupillary abnormalities [1,42]. Levin and colleagues [42] noted that oculovestibular disturbance and duration of coma were related to cognitive impairment on the WAIS. Even when the

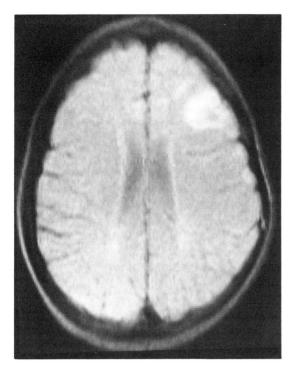

Figure 8.1B. Baseline MRI obtained five days after injury at the identical level as the CT scan shown in Figure 8.1A. A left frontal lesion with heterogeneous signal intensity is disclosed indicating isointense and hyperintense areas relative to the brain. From Levin et al, Magnetic resonance imaging and computerized tomography in relation to the neurobehavioral sequelae of mild and moderate head injuries. Journal of Neurosurgery 66:706-713, 1987. Reprinted with permission of the publisher.

coma durations of patients with or without an oculovestibular deficit were equated, the Verbal IQ was significantly lower in the impaired group, whereas Performance IQ were comparable. Alexandre et al [1] similarly noted that patients with oculovestibular deficits obtained poorer cognitive outcomes. In addition, the best GCS scores documented within 24 hours after admission were predictive of cognitive recovery with 80% of patients who obtained scores of 8 to 15 showing a favorable outcome in contrast to 10% of patients with scores of 3 to 4. Studies have also demonstrated relationships between lateralization of a mass lesion and cognitive functioning. Uzzell et al [80] found that patients with right hemisphere lesions obtained Verbal IQs above those with left hemisphere lesions, whereas Performance IQ differences were nonsignificant. Post-traumatic amnesia, in contrast to these other clinical variables, has been inconsistent as a predictor of long term cognitive outcome [1,52].

One difficulty in analyzing the relationships between clinical indices and intellectual recovery is that the severity variables tend to be intercorrelated and, therefore, the unique contribution of each index is made difficult [37]. In addition, although research has examined return to an "average" level of functioning (e.g., IQs within one standard deviation of the population mean), the extent to which IQ has recovered cannot be determined without a consideration of premorbid levels. Williams and co-workers [85] employed a formula proposed to estimate premorbid IQ on the

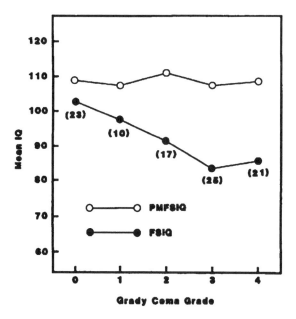

Figure 8.2. The relationship between coma grade and both premorbid (PMFSIQ) and observed Full Scale IQ (FSIQ). Numbers in parentheses represent the number of patients at each coma level. The Grady scale grossly correlates with the Glasgow Coma Scale, but increasing numbers (0 to 5) represent increasing depth of coma. Predicting outcome from closed head injury by early assessment of trauma severity. Journal of Neurosurgery 61:581-585, 1984. Reprinted with permission of the author and publisher. .

WAIS [86] in order to predict intellectual outcome approximately six weeks following CHI. through use of a regression model, the investigators found that post-injury Full Scale IQ was predicted most accurately by the estimated premorbid IQ and coma level (see Figure 8.2), whereas the presence of pupillary abnormality, hemiparesis, and skull fracture was noncontributory. However, the conclusions that can be drawn from this study are limited by an injury-test interval which was too short to assess the full extent of recovery [53]. The increasing use of premorbid estimates and regression models will, we hope, contribute to an understanding of long term outcome.

Reasoning and Problem Solving

The ability to exhibit productive thought and to utilize feedback in order to generate hypotheses or shift strategy is an important, albeit often neglected, component of cognitive functioning. Patients may attain a score within the normal range on a standardized psychometric test of intelligence and yet be markedly impaired in problem solving, regulation of behavior, and planning of activities [74]. Although ablation studies have emphasized the role of the frontal lobes in producing these deficits, neuroanatomic localization in head-injured patients is complicated by the presence of diffuse or multifocal trauma. Levin and colleagues [36] demonstrated the relative advantage of MRI in detecting parenchymal frontal and temporal lesions which were undisclosed by CT scans (See Figure 8.3) in mild or moderately injured patients, confirming the observations of other investigators for the vulnerability of

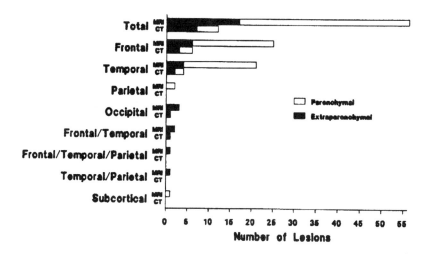

Figure 8.3. Intrahemispheric locus of lesion disclosed by computerized tomography (CT) versus magnetic resonance imaging (MRI) in 20 patients with minor or moderate head injury. From Levin et al, Magnetic resonance imaging and computerized tomography in relation to the neurobehavioral sequelae of mild and moderate head injuries. Journal of Neurosurgery 66:706-713, 1987. Reprinted with permission of the publisher.

these areas [33,61]. The generality of a "frontal lobe" syndrome and the particular sensitivity of tests to focal frontal lobe damage in patients remains to be further established [73].

The Wisconsin [23] and Modified [59] Card Sorting tests may be used to assess deficits in hypothesis testing and ability to benefit from feedback. These procedures require consecutive sorting on one of three dimensions (color, shape, or number) followed by a shift to another dimension. The patient is told after each trial whether or not the response is correct. Patients with frontal lobe damage frequently achieve an impoverished number of correct sorts and tend to make perseverative errors (i.e., to stay with a previously correct principle even though it is not longer reinforced) [56]. Stuss et al [75] examined various aspects of cognitive functioning in head-injured patients with a range of severity who had achieved a good recovery. A good recovery is the highest level of Glasgow Outcome Scale [31]. Despite similarities in performance between patients and controls on tests including intellectual level, patients made an excessive number of perseverative errors on the sorting task.

Another type of deficit is a reduction in productivity such as the generation of responses under timed conditions. Reduced verbal fluency is a feature of left frontal injury [3], whereas diminished capacity to invent novel designs under timed conditions (i.e., reduced design fluency) is a relatively specific finding in patients with right frontal injury [35]. A dissociation in temporal versus frontal lobe lesions on design fluency performance was found by Levin and colleagues [36] with frontal lobe

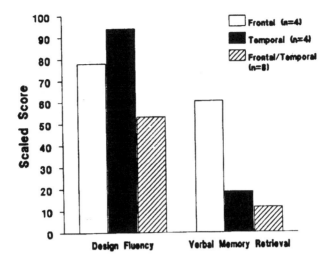

Figure 8.4. Neuropsychological test performance in head-injured patients with focal lesions visualized by magnetic resonance imaging in the frontal and/or temporal regions. To permit direct comparison of design fluency (a measure of frontal lobe functioning) with verbal memory retrieval (a measure primarily of temporal lobe functioning), the performance of the subgroups of patients is plotted as a scaled score in which the mean and standard deviation of the control group are equivalent to 100 and 10, respectively. Accordingly, a scaled score of 100 is equivalent to the mean of the control group while a scaled score of 80 signifies a level of performance that falls two standard deviations below the control group. From Levin et al, Magnetic resonance imaging and computerized tomography in relation to the neurobehavioral sequelae of mild and moderate head injuries. Journal of Neurosurgery 66:706-713, 1987. Reprinted with permission of the publisher.

damaged patients who perseverated. As expected, patients with left frontal lobe lesions exhibited markedly reduced verbal fluency in contrast to those with right frontal lesions.

Memory

A long term memory deficit is frequently present after moderate or severe head injury and may persist in approximately 50% of survivors of severe injury [62,82]. In contrast, although memory impairment is often observed in the initial stages of a mild head injury (i.e., minimal or no loss of consciousness, normal neurologic findings), these problems as measured by objective tests may be resolved by three months in the majority of patients without a previous history of head injury or neuropsychiatric disturbance [12,20,46].

A salient feature of memory after emergence from PTA is difficulty in learning and retaining new information. Populations other than head injury, e.g., epileptic patients undergoing surgery [57,58], have implicated the role of the temporal lobes in contributing to memory disturbance. A disproportionate effect on memory of temporal or frontotemporal lesions following head injury may also occur. As seen in Figure 8.4, patients with lesions confined to these areas exhibited poorer retrieval from long term memory on a test requiring recall of words over multiple trials [11] than those with lesions to the frontal lobes. In contrast, the rapid generation of novel designs, a measure of cognitive flexibility, was relatively preserved in the temporal damaged group.

While temporal lobe lesions may contribute to the manifestation of an initial long term memory deficit in survivors, this effect is relatively transient in contrast to other clinical indices including the degree and duration of impaired consciousness, oculovestibular deficit, and residual ventricular enlargement [1,7,8,37,44]. We recently found that a chronic memory deficit occurs in approximately 25% of survivors of moderate or severe CHI despite intellectual functioning in the average range [39]. The presence of an amnesic disorder (disproportionate impairment of memory with relatively intact IQ) appears related to acute neurologic indices including the presence of nonreactive pupils. Stuss and colleagues [75] noted the increased susceptibility to interference by CHI patients despite obtaining IQs comparable to controls. The increased analysis of dissociations in cognitive functioning and their relation to neurologic indices will be important for planning future rehabilitation efforts.

Recognition memory following moderate injury is characterized by a large number of false positive errors (identifying a new item as previously seen) [27]. However, patients with impaired consciousness lasting 24 or more hours also exhibit difficulty in recognizing recurring pictures. Whereas lesions of the left temporal lobe have been linked to disturbances in retaining verbal material [37], evidence for a specific impairment of nonverbal visual memory in patients with right temporal lesions is less compelling.

Attention

Disturbances involving slow information processing speed and difficulty in focusing and maintaining attention are frequently demonstrated on both subjective and objective measures. Table 8.2, adapted from Gronwall [24], summarizes studies examining the frequency of reports of concentration problems according to severity of injury. As seen, the presence of such complaints exists across the spectrum of patients and appears to abate (although not disappear) in those studies utilizing serial assessments. However, the lack of adequate control groups and early measurement in more severely injured patients complicates interpretation of the relationship between clinical indices and frequency of complaints [24].

Information processing capacity has been examined primarily by the Paced Auditory Serial Addition Test [25,26] which requires the addition of tape-recorded numbers presented at progressively increased speeds. Performance has been found to be initially impaired in patients with mild head injuries but the scores typically

Table 8.2. Incidence of Concentration Problems in Prospective Series of Head-Injury Cases

Authors	Defined by:	N	Months since injury 1	3	6	12	24
Mild injuries							
Lidvall et al [1974]	PTA <24 hr	83	11%	8%	—	—	—
	Control[a]	83	4%	4%	—	—	—
McLean et al [1984]	TOC[b] <24 hr	68	47%	—	—	—	—
Rimel et al [1981]	GCS[c] ≥13	424	—	59%*	—	—	—
Rutherford et al [1977/79]	PTA <24 hr	145	8%	—	—	3%	—
Wrightson et al [1981]	PTA <36 hr	66	—	16%*	—	—	6%*
Moderate to severe injuries							
McLean et al [1984]	TOC[b] 1-6 d	8	75%	—	—	—	—
Rimel et al [1982]	GCS[c] 9-12	170	—	90%*	—	—	—
Van Zomeren & Van den Burg [1985]	PTA 1-7 d	18	—	—	—	—	17%
Severe to very severe injuries							
McKinley et al [1983]	PTA >2 d C[d]	21	—	53%	40%	38%	—
	NC[d]	21	—	26%	40%	9%	—
McLean et al [1984]	TOC[b] >7 d	4	75%	—	—	—	—
Oddy et al [1978]	PTA >24 hr	48	—	—	29%	—	—
Van Zomeren & Van den Burg [1985]	PTA >7 d	39	—	—	—	—	40%

*Asterisk indicates inclusion of memory as well as concentration problems.
[a]Postconcussion-like problems, present before injury.
[b]TOC: time to obey commands.
[c]GCS: Glasgow Coma Scale score [Teasdale and Jennett 1974].
[d]C = cases with compensation claims pending; NC = no claims.
Adapted from Gronwall D, Advances in the assessment of attention and information processing after head injury. In Levin HS, Grafman J, Eisenberg HM (eds), Neurobehavioral Recovery from Head Injury. New York, Oxford University Press, 1987.

improve to the level of controls within one month [25,46]. In contrast, patients with more severe injuries may demonstrate persistent deficits. Levin and colleagues [44] noted the continued impaired performance in information processing rate in a patient with a severe head injury sustained five years earlier.

Reaction time tasks, particularly those involving choices between two or more responses depending upon which stimulus is presented, are also sensitive to the effects of slowed decision processes following CHI. Van Zomeren and Deelman [81] found that longer durations of PTA and coma as well as low GCS scores were associated with slower choice reaction times. Recently, Stokx and Gaillard [72] examined the relationship between reaction time on conventional tests and driving ability in patients two years post-injury who were initially in coma for one to eight weeks. On the driving test, patients were generally as accurate as controls but displayed significantly slower performances in terms of shifting, braking, and dodging cones on a slalom. There was a significant correlation between performance on the laboratory reaction time test and slalom driving time.

Vigilance performance entailing the ability to maintain attention has been relatively unexplored in survivors of head injury. Ewing and colleagues [16] showed that mildly injured patients two years after injury had a vigilance decrement when placed in a hyperbaric chamber that produced hypoxia. The lack of baseline data on this task, however, complicates interpretation of the findings. The inclusion of broad ranges of injury severity and application to real world tasks will increase our knowledge of attentional deficits.

Language Disturbance

Research has indicated the high frequency of language disturbances in survivors of head injury, even in the absence of obvious clinical manifestations. In a study of 125 patients with coma durations ranging from 10 minutes to 6 months who were admitted to a rehabilitation program, Sarno [69] found that all patients manifested some form of processing deficit. Figure 8.5 depicts the language profiles of patients classified according to the severity of their impairments. Thirty percent of the sample demonstrated an aphasic syndrome characterized by expressive and receptive difficulties including impaired naming of common objects and sentence repetition, reduced verbal fluency, and poor auditory comprehension. Thirty-four percent displayed dysarthria coupled with linguistic deficits which were detected only through formal testing. The remaining 36% had a subclinical profile of language deficits on testing without obvious motoric speech problems. Sarno's research points to the importance of formally evaluating language functions and their recovery patterns.

Anomia or word finding difficulty is one of the most salient features of acute aphasia following head injury [29,41,79]. This deficit is often accompanied by verbal paraphasia (substitution of inappropriate words), perseveration and circumlocution with relative preserved comprehension and repetition. Levin et al [41] reported that almost one-half of their sample of acutely injured patients displayed defective naming and reduced verbal fluency. Wernicke's aphasia is another common clinical syndrome characterized by fluent speech but impaired comprehension for auditory and written information and defective repetition which may in part reflect an inability to understand the command [70]. Thomsen [79] also found paraphasias and anomia common in patients who had been in coma for at least 24 hours.

Duration of coma has been an inconsistent predictor of linguistic disturbance in studies which have combined patients with diffuse and focal injuries [e.g., 67,68,69]. Levin and colleagues [43] reported a relationship between coma duration and anomia, writing, and comprehension in patients who were initially aphasic and studied at least 5 months post-injury. Specific language impairments were related to focal left hemisphere damage, whereas more generalized deficits were associated with ventricular enlargement and diffuse swelling. The interhemispheric locus of a

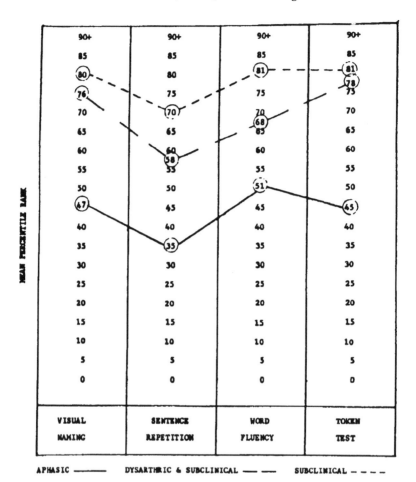

Figure 8.5. Mean percentile rank of aphasic and subclinical language disorder groups on subtests of the Neurosensory Center Comprehensive Examination of Aphasia. From Sarno et al, Characteristics of verbal impairment in closed head injured patients. Archives of Physical Medicine and Rehabilitation 67:400-405, 1987. Reprinted with permission of the author and publisher.

left dominant hemisphere mass lesion appears to be an important correlate of an initial language deficit.

FEATURES OF BEHAVIORAL RECOVERY

The preceding sections have highlighted the salient cognitive dimensions which may be altered following closed head injury. These cognitive changes are frequently accompanied by behavioral manifestations that determine the course and eventual recovery of neurobehavioral functioning. Behavioral disturbances can exaggerate cognitive deficits as in the patient who has a lack of interest towards applying problem-solving skills, or they can stem from neuropsychological impairment as in the patient who appears unmotivated but is actually distractible [63]. In the following sections, we review the common acute and chronic behavioral manifestations and clinicopathological features.

Acute Manifestations

Early manifestations of behavioral change include agitation, inappropriate speech, loss of inhibition, and emotional lability. The presence of initial confusion may be correlated with later disturbances including anxiety and depression, thought disorder, and general psychopathology [40,49]. An antecedent history of neuropsychiatric disorder is not a necessary condition for these features to appear [40]. Questioning the patient may reveal confabulation such as erroneous reasons for being in the hospital as well as paranoid ideation. Visual and auditory hallucinations rarely occur [5,37]. These inappropriate behaviors are often accompanied by disorientation, difficulty in sustaining attention, and impaired memory for daily events (PTA).

The period of acute confusion is typically related to severity of injury. Levin and Grossman [40] found that agitation was associated with initial aphasia and was more prevalent in patients with severe versus mild head injury. However, a subgroup (approximately 10% to 15%) of patients sustaining mild or moderate injuries demonstrate a length of PTA and confusion that is exceedingly prolonged relative to a short duration of impaired consciousness [38]. Although Levin and Grossman [40] did not note an association between agitation and focal lesions based on CT findings, Gandy and colleagues [19] observed that MRI detected areas of edema and contusion (bifrontal, biooccipital, biparietal, and right temporal) missed by CT in a head-injured patient who was agitated, combative, and mute. Whether MRI can elucidate focal hemispheric lesions related to initial behavioral disturbance awaits further study.

Disturbances of Mood

Depression is a frequent affective response following CHI and typically includes alterations in appetite and sleep, energy level, psychomotor responses, and concentration. This reaction is common across the spectrum of severity which may suggest the role of environmental conditions in maintaining the response. Changes in levels of brain catecholamines and cholinergic metabolism may also be important [37]. Studies have indicated persisting depression at times [18,55] despite improvement in other aspects of functioning such as language abilities and behavioral slowing [45].

On the other hand, depression may be accompanied by cognitive deficits, suggesting an interrelationship between personality and neuropsychological components [13].

Other less frequently reported mood disturbances include euphoria characterized by excitable speech and disinhibition. Patients may also display a blunting of affect with lethargy, slow thought processes and passivity as the predominant clinical features. Bilateral lesions of the frontal convexities may be responsible for a "psychodepressed" syndrome in which indifference, apathy, and loss of initiative result. These emotional alterations are often observed in right hemisphere damaged stroke patients [28].

Disturbances of Insight and Motivation

Coupled with changes in mood, patients may fail to appreciate the severity of their deficits, resulting in an impairment of realistic plans and goals. McKinlay and Brooks [54] found that whereas patients and relatives agreed on sensory and motor deficits, they were less likely to concur on emotional and behavioral sequelae with patients tending to minimize their severity. Levin et al [45] found that "metacognition" or knowledge of one's cognitive processes was related to injury severity. Disturbances encompassing self-appraisal (e.g., exaggerated self-opinion, overrating ability in comparison to family and clinicians) and planning (poor formulation of future goals) were common in patients with more severe injuries (GCS ≤ 8). These deficits frequently result from frontal lobe damage [74] although a direct test relating impairments in planning and self-evaluation to frontal lesions following CHI has not been explored.

A disturbance of motivation, another common sequel of CHI, may reflect underlying depression or result from denial of deficits. In addition, brain injury may alter responses to reinforcement, resulting in less effort on the part of the patient to achieve a particular incentive [87]. Social withdrawal, characterized by lessened interactions and engagement in activities, appears to intensify with time [54]. Oddy and Humphrey [60] reported that at one and two years post-injury, 50% of the patients they interviewed participated in fewer activities than before their injuries. Patients with long PTA durations generally had decreased interactions. Moreover, memory disturbance rather than sensory or motor impairments was correlated with reports of fewer friends and social visits.

Somatic Complaints

A third area of change includes somatic complaints such as headaches, dizziness, hypersensitivity to stimuli, and photophobia. These symptoms, coupled with fatigue, irritability, depression, anxiety, decreased concentration and memory, denote the postconcussional syndrome following mild head injury [4]. In a recent three-center study of mild head injury, Levin et al [46] found that complaints involving headaches, decreased energy, and dizziness were still present at three months despite cognitive recovery to the level of control performance. The presence of intracranial lesions undetected by CT, alteration in neurotransmitters, and extracerebral injury may contribute to these symptoms. Pre-injury behavioral features and the post-injury environment must also be considered as determinants.

Van Zomeren and Van Den Burg [82] distinguished between complaints related to severity versus those classified as "intolerances" following severe CHI. PTA duration and return to work correlated with complaints including forgetfulness, slowness, inability to divide attention, and depression. A factor labelled "complaining" was unrelated to PTA and resumption of work and consisted of symptoms such as irritability, fatigue, dizziness, intolerance of light and noise, headaches, and emotional lability. Van Zomeren and Van Den Burg proposed that these latter complaints may develop from stress related to cognitive deficits and expectations of the patient and significant others.

FUTURE AREAS FOR INVESTIGATION

Although our ability to measure and to characterize the neurobehavioral features of closed head injury has advanced over the years, prediction of recovery remains considerably more elusive. Serial investigations employing longitudinal designs and simultaneous examination of a variety of functions will greatly add to this latter task. As the research of Tabaddor and colleagues [76] has shown, neurobehavioral functions recover at differential rates and clinicians may erroneously conclude that further recovery is unexpected based upon an examination one year post-injury. In addition, a unique set of neurological variables may play a role in predicting recovery at different stages. The use of regression equations examining the combination of indices to outcome will be important in contributing to prediction. Moreover, consideration of premorbid features will also be necessary in order to ascertain the extent of recovery.

Studies need to examine the interrelationships and dissociations between aspects of neurobehavioral features. For example, research [39,75] has indicated that while intellectual functioning may be in the average range on formal tests, other components such as memory and problem-solving skills may be selectively impaired. Our knowledge of the relationships between behavioral disturbance and cognitive problems is also sparse. Patients may be overlooked with respect to psychiatric treatment because they lack insight and exhibit an apparent improvement in cognitive ability [5]. Assessment of both psychosocial and cognitive functioning will add to an understanding of patterns of disability.

Frontal lobe dysfunction has been relatively neglected in studies of survivors of closed head injury despite evidence for the vulnerability of frontal regions to damage [33,61]. Clinical observations suggest that decreased motivation, lack of insight, and conceptual disorganization are prominent features in patients [5]. Yet, there has been no direct test to examine whether patients with frontal injury represent a subgroup with special needs for rehabilitation and counselling. Such research would sensitize clinicians to particular problems exhibited by these patients and aid in the design of future remediation strategies.

Finally, many of the studies reported in this chapter have examined relatively young (e.g., age range of 18 to 40) survivors of head injury. There is clearly a need to understand the neurobehavioral effects of head injury in older patients, given the shift in features of our demographic population. Clinicians are currently limited in their ability to predict quality of outcome in these head-injured individuals as well as to understand the remote effects of aging in patients who have been injured at an early point in time.

SUMMARY

The quality of survival after head injury has been more precisely defined in recent years. The Glasgow Outcome Scale (good recovery, modest disability, severe disability, vegetative state) of Jennett and Bond is an excellent indicator of gross outcome by 3 to 6 months after a moderate or severe head injury. However, more subtle neurobehavioral and cognitive changes, often not appreciated by the surgeon or neurologist, may have a devastating impact upon day-to-day functioning of the injured patient, his family and societal contacts. Attempts to identify factors related to recovery will, we hope, improve our ability to predict and treat these disturbances with directed rehabilitation efforts.

The prognostic significance of neurologic indices such as GCS, hemiparesis, brainstem reflexes, focal lesions, and length of PTA are discussed. Features of cognitive recovery—including general intellectual functioning, reasoning, problem solving, memory, attention and language disturbance—as they relate to prognosis and potential for further recovery are reviewed. Accompanying behavioral disturbances unfortunately frequent the above cognitive deficits. Resulting behavior includes confusion, agitation, emotional lability, somatic complaints, and changes in mood, insight, and motivation. Many post-traumatic psychological or behavioral disturbances are related to the severity and focality of injury, the patient's baseline personality, reaction to illness, and an individual's ability to cope with the result of injury. It is hoped that identification of higher function or behavioral problems will lead to a specifically structured cognitive rehabilitative effort for a particular patient. Although the task may be formidable, there is little practical alternative to successful societal reintegration.

ACKNOWLEDGMENTS

Preparation of this chapter was supported in part by the Javits Neuroscience Investigator Award, NS 2-1889, Moody Foundation grant #84-152, and the NIH

National Traumatic Coma Data Bank, NS 3-2339. We thank Liz Zindler for her help in manuscript preparation.

REFERENCES

1. Alexandre A, Colombo F, Nertempi P, Benedetti A. Cognitive outcome and early indices of severity of head injury. J Neurosurg, 1983, 59:751-761.
2. Becker DP, Miller JD, Ward JD, Greenberg RP, Young HF, Sakalas R. The outcome from severe head injury with early diagnosis and intensive management. J Neurosurg, 1977, 47:491-502.
3. Benton AL. Differential behavioral effects in frontal lobe disease. Neuropsychologia, 1968, 12:557-563.
4. Binder LM. Persisting symptoms after mild head injury: A review of the postconcussive syndrome. J Clin Exp Neuropsychol, 1986, 8:323-346.
5. Bond MR. The psychiatry of closed head injury. In: Brooks N (ed), Closed Head Injury: Psychological, Social, and Family Consequences. New York, Oxford Univ Press, 1984.
6. Bond MR, Brooks DN. Understanding the process of recovery as a basis for the investigation of rehabilitation for the brain injured. Scand J Rehab Med, 1976, 8:127-133.
7. Brooks DN. Memory and head injury. J Nerv Ment Dis, 1972, 155:350-355.
8. Brooks DN. Long and short term memory in head injured patients. Cortex, 1975, 11:329-340.
9. Brooks DN. Measuring neuropsychological and functional recovery. In: Levin HS, Grafman J, Eisenberg HM (eds), Neurobehavioral Recovery from Head Injury. New York, Oxford Univ Press, 1987.
10. Brooks DN, Aughton ME, Bond MR, Jones P, Rizvi S. Cognitive sequelae in relationship to early indices of severity of brain damage after severe blunt head injury. J Neurol Neurosurg Psychiat, 1980, 43:529-534.
11. Buschke H, Fuld PA. Evaluating storage, retention, and retrieval in disordered memory and learning. Neurology, 1974, 24:1019-1025.
12. Dikmen S, McLean A, Temkin N. Neuropsychological and psychosocial consequences of minor head injury. J Neurol Neurosurg Psychiat, 1986, 49:1227-1232.
13. Dikmen S, Reitan RM. Emotional sequelae of head injury. Ann Neurol, 1977, 2:492-494.
14. Dikmen S, Temkin N. Determination of the effects of head injury and recovery in behavioral research. In: Levin HS, Grafman J, Eisenberg HM (eds), Neurobehavioral Recovery from Head Injury. New York, Oxford Univ Press, 1987.
15. Drudge OW, Williams JM, Kessler M, Gomes FB. Recovery from severe closed head injuries: Repeat testings with the Halstead-Reitan neuropsychological battery. J Clin Psychol, 1984, 40:259-265.
16. Ewing R, McCarthy D, Gronwall D, Wrightson P. Persisting effects of minor head injury observable during hypoxic stress. J Clin Neuropsychol, 1980, 2:147-155.
17. Fletcher JM, Miner ME, Ewing-Cobbs L. Age and recovery from head injury in children: Developmental issues. In: Levin HS, Grafman J, Eisenberg HM (eds), Neurobehavioral Recovery from Head Injury. New York, Oxford Univ Press, 1987.
18. Fordyce DJ, Roueche JR, Prigatano GP. Enhanced emotional reactions in chronic head trauma patients. J Neurol Neurosurg Psychiat, 1983, 46:620-624.
19. Gandy SE, Snow RB, Zimmerman RD, Deck MD. Cranial nuclear magnetic resonance imaging in head trauma. Ann Neurol, 1984, 16:254-257.
20. Gentilini M, Nichelli P, Schoenhuber R, Bortolotti P, Tonelli L, Falasca A, Merli GA. Neuropsychological evaluation of mild head injury. J Neurol Neurosurg Psychiat, 1985, 48:137-140.

186 *Goldstein, Levin, and Eisenberg*

21. Gilchrist E, Wilkinson M. Some factors determining prognosis in young people with severe head injuries. Arch Neurol, 1979, 36:355-358.
22. Goldstein FC, Levin HS. Intellectual and academic recovery in closed head injured children and adolescents. Dev Neuropsychol, 1986, 1:195-214.
23. Grant DA, Berg EA. A behavioral analysis of degree of reinforcement and ease of shifting to new responses in a Weigl-type card-sorting problem. J Exp Psychol, 1948, 38:404-411.
24. Gronwall D. Advances in the assessment of attention and information processing after head injury. In: Levin HS, Grafman J, Eisenberg HM (eds), Neurobehavioral Recovery from Head Injury. New York, Oxford Univ Press, 1987.
25. Gronwall D, Sampson H. The Psychological Effects of Concussion. Auckland, Auckland Univ Press, 1974.
26. Gronwall D, Wrightson P. Delayed recovery of intellectual function after minor head injury. Lancet, 1974, 2:605-609.
27. Hannay HJ, Levin HS, Grossman RG. Impaired recognition memory after head injury. Cortex, 1979, 15:269-283.
28. Heilman KM, Bowers D, Valenstein E. Emotional disorders associated with neurological diseases. In: Heilman KM, Valenstein E (eds), Clinical Neuropsychology. New York, Oxford Univ Press, 1985.
29. Heilman KM, Safran A, Geschwind N. Closed head trauma and aphasia. J Neurol Neurosurg Psychiat, 1971, 34:265-269.
30. Jenkins A, Teasdale G, Hadley M, MacPherson P, Rowan JO. Brain lesions detected by magnetic resonance imaging in mild and severe head injuries. Lancet, 1986, 2:445-446.
31. Jennett B, Bond M. Assessment of outcome after severe brain damage. Lancet, 1975, 1:480-484.
32. Jennett B, Snoek J, Bond MR, Brooks N. Disability after severe head injury: Observations on the use of the Glasgow Outcome Scale. J Neurol Neurosurg Psychiat, 1981, 44:285-293.
33. Jennett B, Teasdale G. Management of Head Injuries. Philadelphia, FA Davis Co, 1981.
34. Jennett B, Teasdale G, Braakman R, Minderhoud J, Knill-Jones R. Predicting outcome in individual patients after severe head injury. Lancet, 1976, 1:1031-1034.
35. Jones-Gotman M, Milner B. Design fluency: The invention of nonsense drawings after focal cortical lesions. Neuropsychologia, 1977, 15:653-674.
36. Levin HS, Amparo E, Eisenberg HM, Williams DH, High, WM Jr, McArdle CB, Weiner RL. Magnetic resonance imaging and computerized tomography in relation to the neurobehavioral sequelae of mild and moderate injuries. J Neurosurg, 1987, 66:706-713.
37. Levin HS, Benton AL, Grossman RG. Neurobehavioral Consequences of Closed Head Injury. New York, Oxford Univ Press, 1982.
38. Levin HS, Eisenberg HM. Postconcussional Syndrome. In: Johnson RT (ed), Current Therapy in Neurologic Disease. Philadelphia, BC Decker Inc, 1987.
39. Levin HS, Goldstein FC, High WM Jr. Distinction of amnesic disorder versus general cognitive impairment after closed head injury. Presented at the Tenth Annual European Meeting of the International Neuropsychological Society, Barcelona, Spain, July 1987.
40. Levin HS, Grossman RG. Behavioral sequelae of closed head injury. Arch Neurol, 1978, 35:720-727.
41. Levin HS, Grossman RG, Kelly PJ. Aphasic disorder in patients with closed head injury. J Neurol Neurosurg Psychiat, 1976, 39:1062-1070.
42. Levin HS, Grossman RG, Rose JE, Teasdale G. Long-term neuropsychological outcome of closed head injury. J Neurosurg, 1979, 50:412-422.
43. Levin HS, Grossman RG, Sarwar M, Meyers CA. Linguistic recovery after closed head injury. Brain and Language, 1981, 12:360-374.

44. Levin HS, Handel SF, Goldman AM, Eisenberg HM, Guinto FC Jr. Magnetic resonance imaging after "diffuse" nonmissile head injury: A neurobehavioral study. Arch Neurol, 1985, 42:963-968.

45. Levin HS, High WM Jr, Goethe KE, Sisson RA, Overall JE, Rhoades HM, Eisenberg HM, Kalisky Z, Gary HE Jr. The Neurobehavioural Rating Scale: Assessment of the behavioural sequelae of head injury by the clinician. J Neurol Neurosurg Psychiat, 1987, 50:183-193.

46. Levin HS, Mattis S, Ruff RM, Eisenberg HM, Marshall LF, Tabaddor K, High WM Jr, Frankowski RF. Neurobehavioral outcome following minor head injury: A three-center study. J Neurosurg, 1987, 66:234-243.

47. Levin HS, O'Donnell VM, Grossman RG. The Galveston orientation and amnesia test: A practical scale to assess cognition after head injury. J Nerv Ment Dis, 1979, 167:675-684.

48. Lezak MD. Neuropsychological Assessment. New York, Oxford Univ Press, 1983.

49. Lishman WA. Brain damage in relation to psychiatric disability after head injury. Brit J Psychiat, 1968, 114:373-410.

50. Lishman WA. The psychiatric sequelae of head injury: A review. Psychol Med, 1973, 3:304-318.

51. Mandleberg IA. Cognitive recovery after severe head injury, 2: Wechsler Adult Intelligence Scale during post-traumatic amnesia. J Neurol Neurosurg Psychiat, 1975, 38:1127-1132.

52. Mandleberg IA. Cognitive recovery after severe head injury, 3: WAIS verbal and performance IQs as a function of patient amnesia duration and time from injury. J Neurol Neurosurg Psychiat, 1976, 39:1001-1007.

53. Mandleberg IA, Brooks DN. Cognitive recovery after severe head injury, I: Serial testing on the Wechsler Adult Intelligence Scale. J Neurol Neurosurg Psychiat, 1975, 38:1121-1126.

54. McKinlay WW, Brooks DN. Methodological problems in assessing psychosocial recovery following severe head injury. J Clin Neuropsychol, 1984, 6:87-99.

55. McKinlay WW, Brooks DN, Bond MR, Martinage DP, Marsall MM. The short-term outcome of severe blunt head injury as reported by relatives of the injured persons. J Neurol Neurosurg Psychiat, 1981, 44:527-533.

56. Milner B. Effects of different brain lesions on card sorting. Arch Neurol, 1963, 9:100-110.

57. Milner B. Sparing of language functions after early unilateral brain damage. Neurosci Res Prog Bull, 1974, 12:213-217.

58. Milner B. Clues to the cerebral organization of memory. In: Buser PA, Rougeul-Buser (eds), Cerebral Correlates of Conscious Experience. INSERM Symposium No 6. New York, Elsevier North-Holland Biomedical Press, 1978.

59. Nelson HE. A modified card sorting test sensitive to frontal lobe defects. Cortex, 1976, 12:313-324.

60. Oddy M, Humphrey M. Social recovery during the year following severe head injury. J Neurol Neurosurg Psychiat, 1980, 43:798-802.

61. Ommaya AK, Gennarelli TA. Cerebral concussion and traumatic unconsciousness: Correlation of experimental and clinical observations on blunt head injuries. Brain, 1974, 97:633-654.

62. Parker SA, Serrats AF. Memory recovery after traumatic coma. Acta Neurochir, 1976, 34:71-77.

63. Prigatano GP. Personality and psychosocial consequences after brain injury. In: Meier MJ, Benton AL, Diller L (eds), Neuropsychological Rehabilitation. New York, Churchill Livingstone, 1987.

64. Rimel RW, Giordani B, Barth JT, Boll TJ, Jane JA. Disability caused by minor head injury. Neurosurgery, 1981, 9:221-229.

65. Rosenthal M. Behavioral sequelae. In: Rosenthal M. Griffith ER, Bond MB, Miller JD (eds), Rehabilitation of the Head Injured Adult. Philadelphia, FA Davis Co, 1983.

66. Russell WR, Smith A. Post-traumatic amnesia in closed head injury. Arch Neurol, 1961, 5:16-29.

67. Sarno MT. The nature of verbal impairment after closed head injury. J Nerv Ment Dis, 1980, 168:685-692.
68. Sarno MT. Verbal impairment after closed head injury: Report of a replication study. J Nerv Ment Dis, 1984, 172:475-479.
69. Sarno MT, Buonaguro A, Levita E. Characteristics of verbal impairment in closed head injured patients. Arch Phys Med Rehab, 1986, 67:400-405.
70. Sarno MT, Levin HS. Speech and language disorders after closed head injury. In: Darby J (ed), Speech and Language Evaluation in Neurology: Adult Disorders. San Diego, Grune & Stratton Inc, 1985.
71. Shapiro K. Pediatric Head Trauma. New York, Futura Publishing Co Inc, 1983.
72. Stokx LC, Gaillard WK. Task and driving performance of patients with a severe concussion of the brain. J Clin Exp Neuropsychol, 1986, 8:421-436.
73. Stuss DT. Contribution of frontal lobe injury to cognitive impairment after closed head injury: Methods of assessment and recent findings. In: Levin HS, Grafman J, Eisenberg HM (eds), Neurobehavioral Recovery from Head Injury. New York, Oxford Univ Press, 1987.
74. Stuss DT, Benson DF. The Frontal Lobes. New York, Raven Press, 1986.
75. Stuss DT, Ely P, Hugenholtz H, Richard MT, LaRochelle S, Poirier CA, Bell I. Subtle neuropsychological deficits in patients with good recovery after closed head injury. Neurosurgery, 1985, 17:41-47.
76. Tabaddor K, Mattis S, Zazula T. Cognitive sequelae and recovery course after moderate and severe head injury. Neurosurgery, 1984, 14:701-708.
77. Tarsh MJ, Royston C. A follow-up study of accident neurosis. Brit J Psychiat, 1985, 146:18-25.
78. Teasdale G, Jennett B. Assessment of coma and impaired consciousness: A practical scale. Lancet, 1974, 2:81-84.
79. Thomsen IV. Evaluation and outcome of aphasia in patients with severe closed head trauma. J Neurol Neurosurg Psychiat, 1975, 38:713-718.
80. Uzzell BP, Zimmerman RA, Dolinskas CA, Obrist WD. Lateralized psychological impairment associated with CT lesions in head injured patients. Cortex, 1979, 15:391-401.
81. Van Zomeren AH, Deelman BG. Long-term recovery of visual reaction time after closed head injury. J Neurol Neurosurg Psychiat, 1978, 41:452-457.
82. Van Zomeren AH, Van Den Burg W. Residual complaints of patients two years after severe head injury. J Neurol Neurosurg Psychiat, 1985, 48:21-28.
83. Wechsler D. The Wechsler Adult Intelligence Scale Manual. New York, Psychological Corporation, 1955.
84. Wechsler D. WAIS-R Manual. New York, Psychological Corporation, 1981.
85. Williams JM, Gomes F, Drudge OW, Kessler M. Predicting outcome from closed head injury by early assessment of trauma severity. J Neurosurg, 1984, 61:581-585.
86. Wilson RS, Rosenbaum G, Rourke D, Whitman D, Grisell J. An index of premorbid intelligence. J Consult Clin Psychol, 1978, 46:1554-1555.
87. Wood RL. Behavior disorders following severe brain injury: Their presentation and psychological management. In: Brooks N (ed), Closed Head Injury: Psychological, Social, and Family Consequences. New York, Oxford Univ Press, 1984.

Index

189